YOGA FOR MILLENNIALS

YOGA FOR MILLENNIALS

*An ancient practice
for a modern generation*

Shashi K. Agarwal, MD

Also, by author:

- 101 Heart Healthy Lifestyles
  (co-authored with Neil K. Agarwal, MD)
- Negative Notions Positive Potions
  (co-authored with Michael E. Bowman, MSW)
- Emotional Maturity
- Emotional Positivity
- Evidence Based Therapeutic Effects of Yoga
- Evidence Based Health Benefits of Yoga
- Yoga for travelers

First Edition

Disclaimer

This book provides basic yoga exercises. If you have any significant medical issues that prevents you from performing these exercises or if you discomfort doing them – please seek medical permission or advice before embarking on or continuing a self-directed yoga program. Readers should be aware that knowledge of medicine is constantly evolving. This book is not intended as a substitute for the medical advice of your physicians or other trained health care professional.

Do not disregard professional medical advice or delay seeking it because of something you have read in this book. Do not embark on any treatment change without seeking your health care provider's advice. It is a clinician's responsibility, relying on their experience and knowledge of their patients, to determine the best plan of care.

Reviewing or following information contained in this book, does not constitute a physician-patient relationship. The authors and publisher accept no liability for any injury arising out of the use of material contained herein, and make no warranty, express or implied, with respect to the contents of this publication.

Published at CreateSpace Independent Publishing Platform

Printed in the USA

ISBN -13: 978-1987533361

ISBN-10: 1987533364

This book is dedicated to
my son Neil and daughter Ayna
- both millennials

"Plant your garden and decorate your own soul, instead of waiting for someone to bring you flowers."

Jose Luis Borges

CONTENTS

"Do not let the life physically damage you, emotionally disturb you, and spiritually deplete you. Stay in control. With regular exercise, mental positivity and spiritual practice, you can prevent the ravages of 'modern living'. Yoga will help keep you robust, recharged and revitalized."

Shashi K. Agarwal

1. INTRODUCTION

"If every 8-year-old in the world is taught meditation,

we will eliminate violence from the world within one generation."

Dalai Lama

Several millennia ago, astute human ancestors recognized the health benefits of engaging the body in several physical postures – as an exercise. These series of poses were devised by watching living things, especially animals, and many poses are named after them. This knowledge was transferred from generation to generation verbally and via physical illustration. These practices would, after several thousand years, become united under the term 'yoga'.

The term "yoga," is found in ancient India's earliest known scripts — the Vedas. These writings date from the Vedic period, which began in 1500 BCE. They are composed in Vedic Sanskrit and are the oldest writings of Hinduism and Sanskrit literature. The word 'yoga' means 'to join' or 'to yoke' or 'to unite' and is derived from the Sanskrit root 'yuj'. According to the sages, yoga unites the human consciousness with that of the Universal Consciousness. This leads to a perfect harmony between the mind and body, and the humans and nature.

 Patanjali, often considered the father of yoga, systematically organized (approximately 1700 years ago) the ancient knowledge into aphorisms, collectively known as the' Yoga-Sûtras'. Modern yoga is based on these writings. Yoga was introduced to the West in the late 1800s and early 1900s by yoga 'gurus' from India. Swami Vivekananda in the late 19th and early 20th century made an important contribution towards this, but its real popularity in the US started after Indra Devi opened her yoga studio in Hollywood in 1947.

Today, yoga is a popular system of physical exercise across the Western world. The number of yoga practitioners in the US has risen from 4 million in 2001 to 20 million in 2011. And millions more have started practicing yoga across the globe. The medical community has also recognized that yoga practice is associated with a plethora of health benefits. Noting its blossoming popularity, and its evidence-based health benefits, the United Nations General Assembly has marked June 21 as the International Yoga Day.

Health and longevity appears to have peaked in the US. The lifespan has recently shown a downward trend and obesity, inactivity and mental disorders are on the rise. Experts tell us that only about 3% Americans follow a 'healthy' lifestyle. These data do not portend a healthy future for this country. Millennials, the most educated and probably the most health obsessed generation of all times, are unfortunately, travelling along the same road. Besides obesity and inactivity, they are also under considerable emotional stress. It is estimated that 60% of this population is experiencing excessive stress while 51% have depression or anxiety.

Yoga practice can help reverse this negative trend. This book provides a simple 60 pose routine that can be done regularly and can be modified as per time availability. Another set of 30 poses, somewhat intermediate in complexity, are also provided. These can be incorporated into the earlier routine as the practitioner gets comfortable. A set of breathing exercises and meditation techniques are also detailed. These exercises should help keep the practitioner healthy, both physically and mentally, and enhance their spiritual unitedness with the Universal Consciousness.

2. HEALTH WOES OF AMERICA

'Human health is a state of complete physical, mental, and social well-being and not merely the absence of disease or infirmity'.

World Health Organization

In the year 1800, no country had a life expectancy above 40[1]. However, things gradually improved over the next 200 years. In the year 1900, life expectancy (in the USA) for a white male was 47 years and white female was 49 years, while for a black male was 33 years and a black female was 34 years – at birth. In the year 2000, this had increased to 75 and 80 years for whites and 68 and 75 for blacks, respectively[2]. This upward trend however - reversed recently. In 2015, the overall death rate rose 1.2 percent in the US - the first decrease in life expectancy in almost two decades. Death rates rose for white men, white women and black men. They stayed essentially even for black women and Hispanic men and women[3]. Americans are now dying sooner than the residents in many other high-income countries - despite spending far more on health care[4]. Are we in trouble? – probably! One of the major contributors to our declining physical health is our increasing propensity to lead poor lifestyles – a life desperately lacking a prudent diet, optimal body weight and adequate exercise. Smoking, although on the decline, still continues to be a major health factor. It is estimated that less than 3 percent of Americans live a 'healthy lifestyle'[5].

The unhealthy lifestyles have negatively impacted the incidence of several serious diseases[6] including:

- Cardiovascular/cerebrovascular diseases (heart diseases and stroke)
- Cancer (malignant neoplasms)
- Chronic lower respiratory disease
- Accidents (unintentional injuries)
- Alzheimer's disease
- Diabetes mellitus

- Influenza and pneumonia

Cardiovascular diseases (heart diseases and stroke) and cancer are together responsible for more deaths than the next five causes. Cardiovascular disease is a major killer in the United States of America. According to the latest statistics released by the American Heart Association[7] (in 2013) cardiovascular diseases claimed 801,000 lives. Of these, heart disease killed more than 370,000 people and strokes killed nearly 129,000 people. Cardiovascular diseases are even more dangerous in the African-American population - 48 percent of women and 46 percent of men in this group have some form of cardiovascular disease. According to the American Heart Association, about 2,200 Americans die of cardiovascular disease each day - an average of 1 death every 40 seconds. It is estimated that you have one in three chances of dying from cardiovascular disease.

According to the American Cancer Society, it is estimated that in 2017, there will be 688,780 new cancer cases diagnosed and 600,920 cancer deaths in the US[8]. It continues to be the second leading cause of death in the US[9]. Breast cancer is the most common type of cancer in the US, with 268,670 new cases expected in 2018. According to the national breast cancer organization, 1 women is diagnosed with breast cancer every 2 minutes, and 1 woman will die of breast cancer every 13 minutes[10]. The next most common cancers are lung cancer and prostate cancer.

Our mental health has also become deplorable. The American Psychiatric Association reports that in 2015, there were an estimated 43.4 million adults aged 18 or older in the US with a mental illness diagnosed within the past one year[11]. In 2015, it is estimated that 16.1 million adults aged 18 or older in the US had at least one major depressive episode in the past year – representing 6.7% of all US adults[12]. According to the Mental Health Association of America, depression rates in American youth are on the rise[13]. Americans are more stressed today than ever before – according to the American Psychological Association, 57% of all

Americans report as being stressed[14]. Opioid overdoses are also in epidemic proportions in the US - drug overdoses are now the leading cause of death among Americans under age 50[15]. Murders in several major American cities are on track to break records in 2017.[16] Chicago, a major city in the USA, recorded over 630 murders from January 1, 2017 till the end of November 2017. According to data released by Federal Bureau of Investigation[17], during 2015, the USA witnessed approximately 15,696 murders, 90,185 rapes, and 327,374 robberies. Losses due to property crimes were estimated at $14.3 billion.

The 2018 World Happiness Report[18], indicates that Finland is the happiest country in the world, with Norway, Denmark, Iceland, and Switzerland holding the next top positions. USA came at number 18.

Religion has also been declining in the USA - however, spirituality appears to be on the rise. It is estimated that nearly one in three Americans under 35 today are religiously unaffiliated, leading to a decline in church attendance[19]. The rise in spirituality may stem from the increasing doubt on the credibility of religions – partially influenced by astronomical and other scientific discoveries. However, given the plethora of hardships and threats one faces in this modern life, spirituality is often difficult to maintain – or practice.

Millennials also face a health future that appears dismal.

"What lies behind us and what lies before us are small matters compared to what lies within us."

Ralph Waldo Emerson

3. HEALTH STATUS OF THE MILLENNIALS

"The only person you should try to be better than is the person you were yesterday."

Anonymous

Millennials are also known as the Y generation (they follow the X generation) and the i-generation (ipads/iphone etc.). They were born between 1981 and 2000 and constitute the major sector of the US workforce today. They were so named because they were the first to enter the workforce at the dawn of the new millennium (a millennium is 1,000 years.). They were preceded by the Baby Boomers, born between 1946 and 1964 (now entering the retirement age) and the Generation X, born between 1965 and 1980 (this generation faced relative political and economic stability)[1].

Millennials are the most educated generation to date[2] and are estimated to comprise 75% of the global workforce by 2025[3]. The millennial generation view themselves as hard-working and team-oriented[4]. They are more inclined towards online social connectedness and use of technology[5].

Millennials are also struggling with health issues. Almost 21% are still smoking and they are drinking more alcohol than the baby boomers[6]. They are less active - almost two-thirds do not meet recommended guidelines for physical activity[7]. 41% of the millennials are either overweight or obese[8] and the levels of obesity are continuing to rise in this population[9]. They do not eat the recommended amount of fruits and vegetables[10]. Their psychological health is also not that good[11]:

- 53 percent of millennials complain of poor sleep.
- Depression or anxiety affects 51 percent of millennials.
- 60 percent millennials report excessive stress.
- 39 percent millennials have self-doubt

Their personal relationships are also not that healthy. According to Chen, author of 'Hellen Chen's Love Seminar Book' over 85% of dating ends up in breakups.[12] And about 40 percent of marriages end in divorce.[13]

They tend to have lower productivity[14] and often earn less than the previous generations at the same age - today 70 percent of minimum wage workers are millennials[15]. They are saddled with high levels of credit and student loan debts, and are therefore unable to save for the future (>95% saving inadequately)[16]. Almost 66% of millennials have nothing saved for their retirement[17].

They are less likely to have health insurance[18] and only 61% see a primary care physician[19]. And as they get older and reach middle age – they are starting to adopt more detrimental life-styles – making them more prone to cardiovascular/cerebrovascular diseases (heart diseases and stroke) and cancer (malignant neoplasms). However, they are more open to utilizing alternative health-care modalities. It is estimated that 64% of millennials perform specific activities to achieve mindfulness, like yoga and meditation[20].

Yogic lifestyle and yogic exercises as described in this book will help prevent, delay the onset of, diminish the severity of or even reverse many of the major diseases mentioned above.

4. HEALTH BENEFITS OF YOGA

"Treatment originates outside; healing comes from within."

Andrew Weil

Yoga practice induces profound measurable physiologic changes in the human body – literally affecting every biochemical and neurological action at a cellular level – leading to helpful changes in normal and diseased individuals[1]. Multimodal yoga (asanas, pranaymas and dhyana) involved biological effects (somewhat scientific) and benefits include:

• There is an improvement in the strength (especially of the core muscles) and flexibility[2]. Endurance is enhanced[3]. Balance[4] and co-ordination is improve[5].

• Respiratory (lung) parameters, such as forced vital capacity, forced expiratory volume during the first second (FEV1), FEV1/FVC ratio, forced expiratory volume during the middle one half of the FVC (FEV 25-75%), peak expiratory flow rate (PFR), maximum voluntary ventilation (MVV) and slow vital capacity, improve[6-9]. These improvements indicate better lung capacity and function. The muscles of respiration are strengthened[10].

• There is an improvement in cardiovascular parameters. There is a decrease in blood pressure[11]. and peripheral arterial resistance[12]. Lipid profile is improved[13]. There is an increase in ejection fraction[14], cardiac output[15] and heart rate variability (better heart function)[16]. There is a decrease in coronary atherosclerosis (decreases risk of heart attack)[17].

• There is a down-regulation of the hypothalamo-pituitary-adrenal (HPA) axis with decreased cortisol levels (stress hormone)[18,19], and increased neurotransmitter gamma-aminobutyric acid (GABA) levels[20]32. Increased GABA levels help improve the mood[21,22].

• Serotonin levels are increased. (serotonin positively affects the mood)[23]. Yoga may also increase endogenous dopamine release in the ventral striatum, a major area of the brain's reward system, explaining the 'feel good' reward with yoga[24]. Oxytocin levels improve, especially in schizophrenics – oxytocin improves social cognition abilities[25].

•   There is an increase in the grey matter in the prefrontal cortex (improved function of the executive center)[26,27], and hippocampus (with a decrease in neuro-senescence – neurological aging)[28] and a decrease in the volume of amygdala (resulting in a decrease in anxiety and fear)[29]. Executive function, including cognition is improved[30,31]. There is more self-awareness and self-regulation. Neuroplasticity within the brain, especially between the basal ganglia, thalamus and cortex occurs, allowing for a better top-down control.

•   Meditation helps reduce mind wandering and negative rumination. There is an increased self-compassion and self-transcendence. Meditation practices have also been shown to increase melatonin levels[32], brain derived neurotrophic factor levels[33] and improve cognitive processes[34]. Meditation results in increased regional blood flow to the prefrontal cortex and anterior cingulate gyrus[35] (and a change in the electrical activity of the brain with more alpha and theta waves (indicating a non-stressful state)[36].

•   Sympathetic activity (flight or fight – stressful for the body) is decreased. Levels of plasma epinephrine and norepinephrine (catecholamines secreted from adrenal medulla) are decreased following yogic practice[37].

•   Parasympathetic activity (rest and digest – good for the body) is increased[38-41]. This increase in parasympathetic activity, primarily with vagus stimulation, improves the bottom-up control.

•   Biomarkers of inflammation are reduced[42-44]. Inflammation is a critical factor behind the development and progression of atherosclerosis[45] and possibly cancer[46].

•   There is an increase in the left insular grey and white matter, with yoga practice. This correlates with increased pain tolerance [47]. Immune function is also improved[48].

•   Overall quality of life is improved[49].

No wonder, more than two-thirds of yoga practitioners report that yoga improved their overall health. Nearly, two-thirds reported that because of practicing yoga they were motivated to exercise more regularly, and 4 in 10 reported they were motivated to eat healthier. More than 80 percent of yoga users reported reduced stress with yoga[50]. Most felt better – they reported a greater sense of relaxation, improved body-image and self-confidence, increased attentiveness, enhanced efficiency, lower irritability, improved interpersonal relationships, and a more positive and optimistic outlook on life. Benefits noted in healthy people include[51] :

General Health:

Cardiovascular:

- Heart disease incidence and complications decrease. It helps reduce your blood pressure.
- The heart rate slows down.
- Cholesterol profile improves, bad cholesterol levels decline.
- Weight declines to a better level.
- Inflammation is reduced
- Blood is thinned.

Pulmonary:

- Respiration is slower, deeper and calmer.
- Respiratory parameters improve – there is an increase in breathing volumes and capacity.
- Breath holding capacity improves. The respiratory stamina increases.
- All respiratory muscles – primary and secondary are exercised.
- Gas exchange in the lung alveoli improves.
- Gas exchange at the cellular level improves.
- Improves nasal breathing.

Neurological:

- Brain function improves. There is better synchronicity between the two brain hemispheres; creativity improves.
- Pain levels decrease.
- Parasympathetic activity (rest and digest) improves while sympathetic activity (flight or fight) declines – the nervous system is more balanced and more relaxed.

Musculo-skeletal:

- Muscle strength increases.
- Coordination is better. There is better depth perception, improved dexterity and better steadiness.
- Flexibility improves.
- Range of motion improves.
- Posture/balance improves.
- Joint health improves.

Other systems:

- Gastrointestinal function improves.
- Urinary excretion is facilitated.
- Immunity increases.
- Endocrine function improves.
- Sexuality improves.
- There is greater relaxation (galvanic skin response improves).
- Addiction, violent and self-destructive behavior decreases.

Quality of life:

- Energy levels go up.
- Sleep is better
- Self-acceptance/self-confidence improves.
- Academic scores go up. Work performance improves.
- Happiness levels rise.

- Health improves - there are less physician visits.
- Life expectancy goes up.
- Your overall quality of life improves.

Spirituality:

- Person becomes more empathic and compassionate.
- There is development of a deeper sense of meaning and purpose to life.
- Overall spirituality increases.

Yoga also gives the benefit of exercise and can help you meet the recommended leisure time activity requirements. The 2008 Physical Activity Guidelines for Americans[52] recommend that children and adolescents get 60 minutes of exercise daily. Exercise should include moderate to vigorous aerobic physical activity daily with muscle-strengthening physical activity on at least 3 days of the week and bone-strengthening physical activity on at least 3 days of the week. Adults should get 150 minutes (2 hours and 30 minutes) a week of moderate-intensity, or 75 minutes (1 hour and 15 minutes) a week of vigorous-intensity aerobic physical activity plus muscle-strengthening activities that are moderate or high intensity and involve all major muscle groups on 2 or more days a week.

Physical activity or physical exercise is measured in METs (Metabolic Equivalent). One MET is approximately equal to a person's resting energy expenditure (e.g. sitting quietly in a chair)[53]. Physical activity is categorized into three categories: light-intensity activities are defined as 1.1 MET to 2.9 METs; moderate-intensity activities are defined as 3.0 to 5.9 METs and vigorous-intensity activities are defined as 6.0 METs or more[54].

Larson-Meyer[55] reviewed 17 studies and concluded that METs for yoga practice averaged 3.3 ± 1.6. METs for individual asanas averaged 2.2 ± 0.7– low to moderate intensity, whereas that of pranayamas was 1.3 ± 0.3 – low intensity. Yoga is therefore generally considered as a light intensity exercise[56,57]. Energy expended during sun salutations depends on the intensity of practice. The estimated METs for sun salutations ranges from 2.9 (light intensity) to 7.4 (vigorous)[55]. High speed sun salutations therefore meet the criteria for vigorous exercise, both in adults[58] and children[59]. Sun salutations in hot atmosphere burns the same number of calories as in thermos-neutral atmosphere[60]. Besides being dynamic, sun salutations also involve static and stretching phases, and exercise most major muscles and joints[61].

Medical Disorders:

The physical and mental health benefits of yoga have undergone human testing and confirmation, although unscientifically, over thousands of years in millions of common people. Its survival over the centuries and its continued (and increasing) acceptance by the human society attests to its beneficial nature. Recently, yogic practices have also been subjected to aggressive and extensive scientific scrutiny, and most of the touted benefits have received an evidence-based nod from the health professionals. Yoga is increasingly being shown to not only to be good for health maintenance - it is also a great preventive and often a 'high value' complementary therapeutic modality.

Research studies on yoga and medical conditions published in 2013 were three times as high as in 2010[62]. The most common research publications on yoga and medical conditions were related to breast cancer, depression, asthma, and type 2 diabetes mellitus[62]. There were also significant number of studies on low back pain and hypertension. Yoga has always been a multimodal practice[63] (combination of postures, breathing exercises and meditation). Some researchers have also included lectures on yoga-based philosophy. Besides the therapeutic benefits noted in specific conditions, yoga has also demonstrated a major benefit on improving the quality of life in these patients[64]. Most of the emerging data is painting a favorable picture of yoga as an adjunct therapeutic modality in several common diseases.

Medical disorders where yoga has shown benefit[65] include: alcoholism, anxiety. asthma, ADHD, back pain, cancer, carpel tunnel syndrome, COPD, coronary artery disease, congestive heart failure, depression, diabetes mellitus, drug addiction, eating disorders, epilepsy, fibromyalgia, heart diseases, heart attack rehabilitation, high blood pressure, HIV/AIDS, infertility, insomnia, irritable bowel syndrome, menopausal disorders, migraine, multiple sclerosis, obsessive compulsive disorder, osteoarthritis, osteoporosis, pain, post-op recovery, post-stroke rehabilitation, pregnancy related disorders, rheumatoid arthritis, rhinitis, schizophrenia, scoliosis and urinary incontinence. The adjunct value of yoga in many other diseases is being studied.

"Yoga is the journey of the self, through the self, to the self."

The Bhagavad Gita

5. WHAT IS YOGA?

"Yoga is a benevolent friend that is always there to greet you with a smile."

David Swenson

Yoga, a form of 'holistic' exercise cum relaxation technique. As practiced in the West, multimodal yoga usually incorporates three processes: postures, breathing exercises and meditation. Most yoga sessions last about an hour and despite the exercise, are relaxing and invigorating. Yoga has become extremely popular in the United States. According to the National Center for Complimentary and Integrative Health[1], 9.5% of U.S. adults (21 million) used yoga and 3.1% of U.S. children (1.7 million) used yoga in 2016. This is a significant increase from 5.1% in 2002 and 6.1% in 2007. According to Yoga Journal and Yoga Alliance, there may be over 30 million yoga practitioners in the USA today. (Yoga Journal) In 1997, only 400,000 health clubs offered yoga classes, but in 2002, over 1.2 million health clubs offered yoga classes[2].

Yoga is extremely old – it has probably been around for about 5000 years. About 1700 years ago, Pantanjali, penned eight limbs of yoga, in 'Yoga sūtras' (sutra = a rule or aphorism), a text on Yoga theory and practice. These are:

- Yama – Morality. Yamas are further classified into five limbs:

    Ahimsa: nonviolence toward all living things. Kindness and compassion to all.

    Satya: being truthful – being always transparent.

    Asteya: non-stealing. You do not mentally or physically take something that is not yours.

    Brahmacharya: celibacy – or proper use of sexual energy.

Aparigraha: the virtue of non-possessiveness, non-grasping or non-greediness. It also encompasses non-attachment.

- Niyama – Personal observances –also five in number:

    Sauca: outer and inner cleanliness. This includes physical as well as mental cleanliness.

    Santosa: contentment – finding happiness in whatever we have. Not longing for what we do not have.

    Tapas: discipline – in life, and in everything we do.

    Svadhyaya: self-inquiry, self-realization. Becoming aware of one's limitations.

    Isvarapranidhana: establishing spirituality – a connection with a higher power.

- Asana – Body movement, physical postures.

- Pranayama – Control of 'prana' (prana = cosmic energy) through controlled breathing.

- Pratyahara – Sense control through sensory withdrawal.

- Dharana – Concentration of the mind.

- Dhyana – Meditation.

- Samadhi – Union with the divine.

As mentioned earlier, the multi-modal yoga practiced in the West includes postures, breathing exercises and meditation. Multi-modal yoga is a low-impact, low-intensity exercise[3]. It is simple and easy to do[4]. It is non-competitive. It can be practiced in a non-secular way[5]. It can be done by all communities, irrespective of the race or income[6-8]. Its practice is feasible in both physically disabled[9] and mentally disabled people[10]. It can also be done by low vision or blind people[11]. It is non-pharmacological and non-surgical. It does not require any special equipment – except maybe a mat. It can however be done without a mat – on a carpet, the grass or sand[12]. It can be individually tailored, especially for the seniors[13]. It is inexpensive and is a potential attractive cost-effective adjunct to more traditional medical therapies. (compared to pharmaceutical or surgical interventions and when done at home). Serious complications are rare[14]. It can be done at any time, including during working hours[15]. Its practice is possible in all age groups[16-19]. Adherence is good[20] with only a few drop outs. One study in adults reporting an attrition rate of only 16%[21]. This compares to an attrition rate of 30% in a study which involved walking and balance exercises[22]. Increasing scientific evidence, also confirms its feasibility in most medical conditions[23].

Yoga has no known interactions with prescription medications[24]. It can be practiced anywhere – home, club, airport, hotel, office – even in prison[25,26]. Healthy yoga practitioners also tend to practice healthy lifestyles: Levels of obesity (4.9%), smoking (2%), and fruit and vegetable consumption are favorable in yoga practitioners when compared to national norms[27]. Healthy yoga practitioners reported that the more yoga they did, the healthier they felt[27]. Length of lifetime yoga practice was significantly associated with better physical health, suggesting yoga has a potential cumulative benefit over time[28]. Emerging scientific data strongly indicates that healthier lifestyles have the potential to increase the human life span by as much as 7-12 years.

"The body is your temple. Keep it pure and clean for the soul to reside in."

B.K.S Iyengar

6. YOGA PRACTICE: BASIC INSTRUCTIONS

*"Nothing would be done at all if we waited until we could do it
well that no one could find fault with it."*

Cardinal Newman

This yoga guide discusses practical performance of asanas,
pranayamas and dhyana – the whole process should take about an
hour. Use a yoga mat, a clean sheet and a flat comfortable site –
any room, deck or even the grass outside. Wear comfortable
clothes and carry a mat or towel with you. The approximate
timings (Sequence I) are as follows: Asana (60 poses): 30 minutes;
Pranayama: 10 minutes; Dhyana: 5 minutes. Total time for yoga
session: approximately 45 minutes) Sequence II includes 30 more
poses and additional breathing and meditation exercises and may
take about 80-90 minutes. Practice this sequence – for a better
flow and comfort. Yoga should ideally be done at least 3 times a
week. Even if you do it once a week, it will still be beneficial to
your health. Breathing exercises can also be done even at night
before sleeping or on waking up. Some forms of meditation – such
as meditative visualization and meditative affirmations, can be
done anytime and anywhere.

Precautions:

Asanas: Although yoga asanas are safe, some precautions are
needed:

- Movement during each pose and during transition should
  be slow and smooth.
- Timed inhalation, timed exhalation and normal breathing
  during hold or transitions should remain smooth and even.
  However, the breathing advice and timings are just a rough
  guidance. Adjust breathing patterns and timings according
  to your convenience. However, hold phase should be for at
  least 10 seconds.
- You will be able to do yoga better on an empty stomach.

- Try to shut off your awareness of all external stimuli during the practice – your ears are open, but you do not hear anything, your eyes are open, but you do not notice anything – and so on.
- Do not exceed your current ability, even if otherwise healthy. You will find that your ability will gradually increase with continuing practice.
- Limit your stretch, gaze or hold if suffering from restrictive joint diseases like arthritis.
- Limit your postures and timings if you have high blood pressure or heart disease – get clearance from your health care provider first.
- If you feel dizzy, pain, or any other uncomfortable sensation, come out of the pose, rest and get some medical advice before continuing again.
- If you have a medical problem requiring medications, you may want to get an approval from your private physician or health care professional.
- Do not stop taking any medications.
- And finally, do not break any local rules - whenever you are performing yoga on the go.

Pranayama:

- The room should be well ventilated – if possible. Ideally do these exercises outside in a natural setting.
- The best time to do these exercises is in the morning.
- You should be wearing loose clothes.
- Do asanas first before proceeding to pranayama exercises.
- Do not do breathing exercises on a full stomach – ideally wait 3-5 hours after eating.
- Always breathe through the nose, unless otherwise instructed.
- Breathing exercises should be comfortable and without any strain.
- Breathing should be quiet – without any loud sounds.

- Normal breathing should be calm and rhythmic. Rapid breathing is akin to hyperventilation and can lead to dizziness.
- Breath holding is often difficult and should be practiced only if comfortable.
- If you find difficulty doing pranayama in the sitting position, try the *savasana* pose.
- Do not perform these exercises if your nose is congested or blocked.
- If you have medical conditions for which you take medications (especially heart or lung diseases) – get clearance from a health care provider before proceeding with these exercises.
- If you feel short of breath or otherwise uncomfortable, stop the exercises and rest in the *savasana* pose.
- Pranayama exercises should be followed by 5 or more minutes of rest – or meditation.

Dhayana:

- Meditation requires a comfortable pose and a quiet atmosphere.
- Meditation gets better as you practice. Do not get frustrated if your mind wanders.
- If you doze off – it is ok. The nap will do you good.

"Yoga is a light, which once lit, will never dim. The better your practice, the brighter the flame."

B.K.S lyengar

7. SEQUENCE I

a. Asanas

Asanas are physical postures. Although I have mentioned their Sanskrit names (in *italics*), you do not have to remember them. I find that the best sequence not only covers all major joint/bone and muscle groups, but also flows gradually, from the start to the relaxation phase – and takes about 30 minutes to do (approximately 30 seconds per pose).

This sequence, that I teach, is as follows:

1. **Standing Poses**: These are grounding postures. While standing on your feet, your spine and body is aligned, and the center of gravity is in the middle. These poses create strength in your legs, allow spinal movements in all directions including twisting, while anchoring your hips. They help create stability and improve coordination.

2. **Kneeling/Seated Poses**: These work on opening the adductor muscles of the hips and improve flexibility of the lower back and spine. These muscles and bones get stretched, toned and relaxed.

3. **Prone Poses**: These are done lying face down, on your stomach. These work on the shoulders and back muscles.

4. **Supine Poses**: These poses are done with face up and lying on the back. These help you work on your upper front chest and abdominals, shoulders and back muscles. The supine pose is also conducive to total body relaxation, natural breathing and meditation.

These exercises will also strengthen your 'core' muscles – and make you develop a good posture and strong balance.

REST POSITIONS:

Whenever you need a break - muscle fatigue, ligament discomfort, breathing with difficulty or having the pose uncoordinated or erroneous - or you just want to take a break, use the following rest positions:

1. Standing: Mountain Pose *(Tadasana)*

2. Sitting: Hero Pose and Easy Pose *(Sukhasana),* Child Pose *(Balasana)*

3. Prone: Sphynx Pose *(Salamba Bhujangasana)*

4. Supine: Corpse Pose *(Savasana)*

The following asanas should be ideally done in the sequence listed. Each pose flows into the next pose. However, once you get comfortable in the poses, you may vary them according to your time and liking. Remember though, the process of transition between postures should be smooth and non-jerky. You should strive for mental and physical stillness during the hold phase, with quiet and easy breathing through your nostrils. The Sanskrit names are given in *italics* and are just for reference. The Sanskrit names have been occasionally modified by me.

SUN SALUTION

Eleven poses done one after another – with each pose coinciding with one half of the breath. These are considered fast yoga routines and are moderate in intensity. They help warm up the body – and burn calories. They can also be done by themselves – without any follow-up with the slow routine or breathing exercises and meditation.

1. Start: Mountain pose *(Tadasana)*
2. Inhalation: Upward salute pose *(Urdhva Hastasana)*
3. Exhalation: Deep forward fold *(Uttanasana)*
4. Inhalation: Standing half forward bend *(Ardha Uttanasana)*

5. Exhalation: Four limbed staff pose *(Chaturanga andasana)*
6. Inhalation: Upward facing dog *(Urdhva Mukha Svanasana)*
7. Exhalation: Downward facing dog *(Adho Mukha Svanasana)*
8. Inhalation: Standing half forward bend *(Ardha Uttanasana)*
9. Exhalation: Deep forward fold *(Uttanasana)*
10. Inhalation: Upward salute *(Urdhva Hastasana)*
11. Exhalation: Back to Mountain pose *(Tadasana)*

These are described in more details later in this chapter.

SEQUENCE OF 60 POSES

STANDING POSES

1. Mountain Pose *(Tadasana)*
2. Upward Salute *(Urdhva Hastasana)*
3. Standing half forward bend *(Ardha Uttanasana)*
4. Modified Mountain Pose *(Modified Tadasana)*
5. Crescent Moon in Mountain Pose *(Ardha Chandrasana)*
6. Deep Forward Bend *(Uttanasana)*
7. Right Leg Forward Bend Both Hands *(Trikonsana variation)*
8. Left Leg Forward Bend Both Hands *(Trikonsana variation)*
9. Wide Legged Mountain *(Utthita Tadasana)*
10. Both Hands to Right Big Toe Pose *(Utthita Trikonasana)*
11. Both Hands to Left Big Toe Pose *(Utthita Trikonasana)*
12. Crescent Moon in Wide Legged Mountain Pose *(Ardha Chandrasana)*
13. Forward Bend with palms on floor *(Prasarita Padottanasana)*
14. Side Bend in Wide Legged Mountain Pose: Right Side *(Utthita Parsvakonasana)*
15. Side Bend in Wide Legged Mountain Pose: Left Side *(Utthita Parsvakonasana)*
16. Warrior I: *(Virabhadrasana I)* Right Foot Forward - Right Knee Bent

17. Forward High Lunge in Warrior I (*Utthita Ashwa Sanchalanasana)* Right Foot Forward - Right Knee Bent
18. Reverse Warrior (*Viparita Virabhadrasana)* with Right Foot Forward - Right Knee Bent
19. Warrior I: (*Virabhadrasana I)* Left Foot Forward - Left Knee Bent
20. Forward High Lunge in Warrior I *(Utthita Ashwa Sanchalanasana)* - Left Foot Forward - Left Knee Bent
21. Reverse Warrior (*Viparita Virabhadrasana)* with Left Foot Forward
22. Warrior II (*Virabhadrasana II)* with Right Knee Bent - Twist Right and hold and then Left
23. Warrior II (*Virabhadrasana II)* with Left Knee Bent - Twist Left and hold and then Right
24. Standing Chair (*Utkatasana)*

KNEELING/SITTING POSES

25. Garland (*Malasana)*
26. Hero Pose (*Virasana)*
27. Easy Pose (*Sukhasana)*
28. Butterfly (*Baddha Konasana)*
29. Staff Pose (*Dandasana)*
30. Half Bound Forward Bend - Right Leg Straight Ardha Baddha (*Padma Pashimottanasana* - variation)
31. Half Bound Forward Bend - Left Leg Straight Ardha Baddha (*Padma Pashimottanasana* - variation)
32. Thunderbolt Pose (*Vajrasana)*
33. Crescent Moon in Hero Pose (*Ardha Chandrasana in Vajrasana)*
34. Child Pose (*Balasana)*
35. Extended Puppy Pose (*Uttana Shishosana)*
36. Standing Thunderbolt Pose (Standing *Vajrasana)*
37. Gate Latch: Right Leg Extended (*Parighasana)*
38. Gate Latch: Left Leg Extended (*Parighasana)*
39. Downward Facing Dog (*Adho Mukha Svanasana)*
40. Low Lunge: Lizard: Right Knee Front and Bent (*Anjaneyasana)*
41. Low Lunge: Lizard: Left Knee Front and Bent (*Anjaneyasana)*

LYING FACE DOWN POSES

42. Sphynx (*Salamba Bhujangasana*)
43. Dolphin Plank (*Makara Adho Mukha Svanasana*)
44. Cobra (*Bhujangasana*)
45. Upward Facing Dog (*Urdhva Mukha Svanasana*)
46. Downward Facing Plank (*Kumbhakasana*)
47. Locust (*Salabhasana*)
48. Bow (*Dhanurasana*)
49. Reclining Buddha: Right Side (*Mahaparinirvanasana*)
50. Side Plank: Right Side (*Vasisthasana*)
51. Reclining Buddha: Left Side (*Mahaparinirvanasana*)
52. Side Plank: Left Side (*Vasisthasana*)

LYING FACE UP POSES

53. Corpse Pose (*Savasana*)
54. Boat (*Navasana*)
55. Happy Baby Pose (*Ananda Balasana*)
56. Wind Relief Pose (*Pawanmuktasana*)
57. Bridge Pose (*Setu Bandha Sarvangasana*)
58. Upward Plank (*Purvottanasana*)
59. Supine spinal twist – revolved abdominal pose: Right Side (*Jathara Parivartanasana*)
60. Supine spinal twist – revolved abdominal pose: Left Side (*Jathara Parivartanasana*)

Final: Corpse pose (#53) (*Savasana*) with Supine stretch (*Supta uttanasana*) to *Savasana*.

Once you feel comfortable with the above routine, you may want to incorporate the 30 more asanas (*with sanskrit names*) – interspersed in the first routine. These are described after the details of Sequence I. The pictures and 'how to' on these 30 extra postures follows the first 60 postures.

Getting into the pose should be smooth and gentle and take about 3-5 seconds. Each pose is held for 10 seconds (or more) or to a slow count of 10 (one-Mississippi, two-Mississippi onwards). Getting out of pose should again be smooth and gentle (no jerking movements) and take about 3-5 seconds. Each transition period is for about 5 seconds. Again, these are only rough guidelines. Try to maintain the final 'hold' for 10 seconds or more depending upon your ability. Remember – there should be no stress.

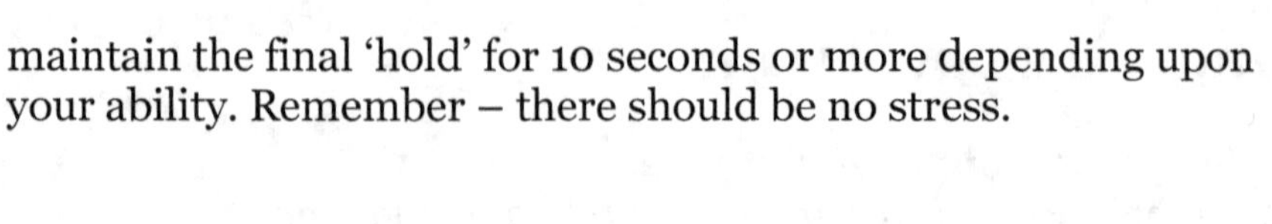

"The body benefits from movement, and the mind benefits from stillness."

Sakyong Mipham

Sun Salutation
(Clockewise from the top)

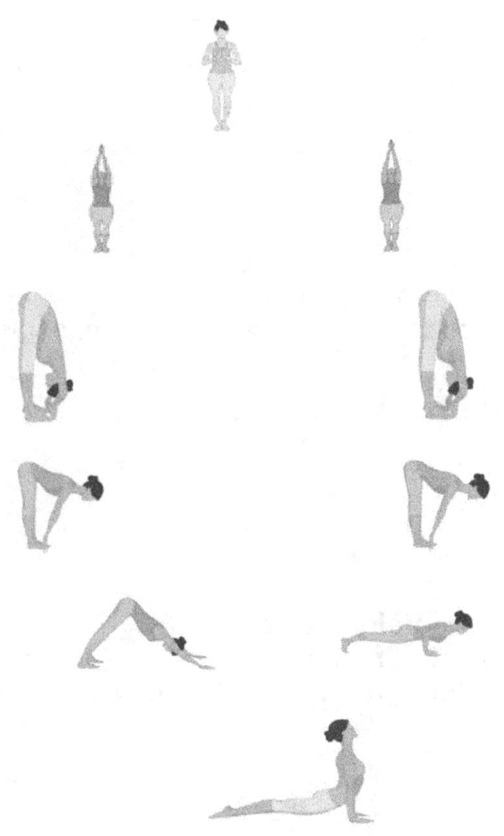

Move through this sequence quickly – one pose during inhalation and one pose during exhalation. This sequence is stimulating and will warm you up quickly. Start with 6 repetitions and gradually build to 12 repititions. These can be done at the start of the slow yoga sequence or independently anytime during the day.

1. Standing Mountain Pose — *Tadasana*
Stand with your feet slightly apart. Press your palms together in prayer position (*Anjali* mudra). Your thumbs should be touching your sternum and fingers pointing up. Yor should be relaxed.

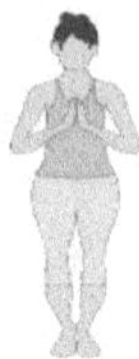

2. Upward Salute — *Urdhva Hastasana*
Inhale as you lift your arms out to the side and overhead. Press the palms against each other. Arch your back gently and look upwards.

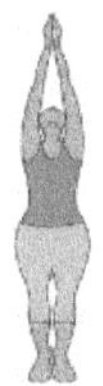

3. Standing Forward Fold — *Uttanasana*
Exhale as you fold forward from the hips. Try to reach the toes with your hands and touch the knees with your nose. Go only as far as you can go comfortably.

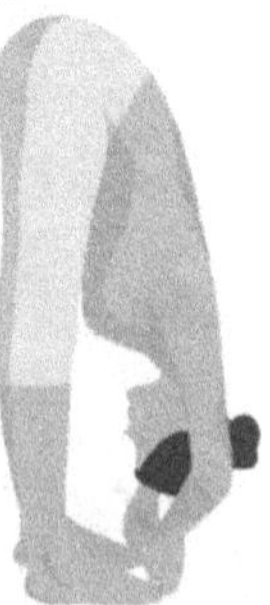

4. Half Standing Forward Fold — *Ardha Uttanasana*
Inhale as you lift your torso halfway and parallel to the floor. Your hands should be touching your feet or your shins.

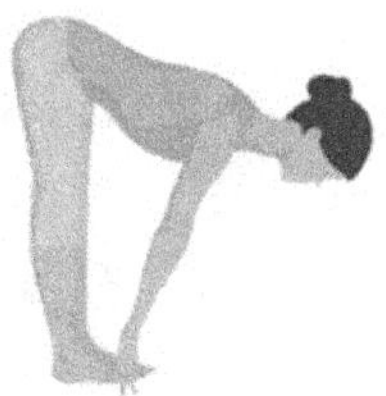

5. **Four-Limbed Staff Pose** — *Chaturanga Dandasana*
Exhaling lower your body towards the floor. Stretch yourself so that you are body is parallel to the floor and you are resting on your toes and palms. The palms should be flat on the floor and you are looking at the floor in front of you. Your wrists and elbows are in one line.

6. **Upward-Facing Dog Pose** — *Urdhva Mukha Svanasana*
Inhaling, lift your upper chest towards the sky. Your arms will become straight and the wrists, elbows and shoulder are now in one line. Your thighs should be off the floor. The elbows are touching the sides of the body.

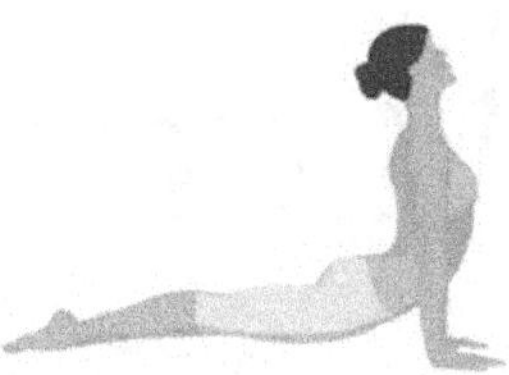

7. **Downward-Facing Dog Pose** — *Adho Mukha Svanasana*
Exhaling, lift your hips and move the soles of the feet on the floor. As you get into the pose, the heels may move off the floor. Stretch your arms forwards, with the palms on the floor, as you arch the back upwards. Your sitting end should be the highest point facing the ceiling/sky.

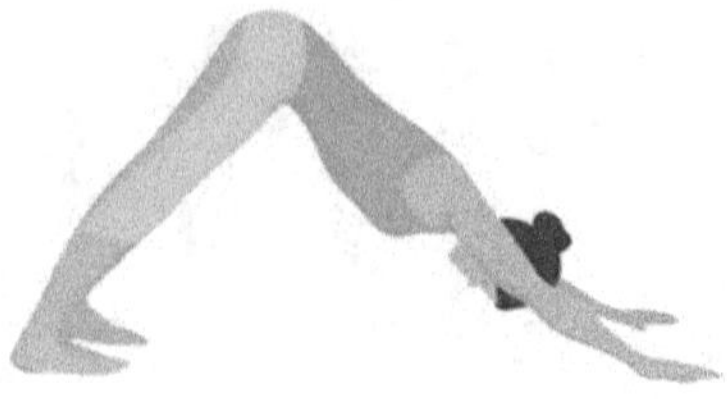

8. **Half Standing Forward Fold** — *Ardha Uttanasana*

Inhale as you lift your torso halfway, so that it becomes parallel to the floor. Bring your fingertips to your feet or your shins. You are looking at your feet.

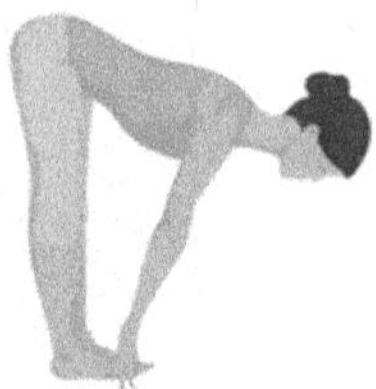

9. **Standing Forward Fold** — *Uttanasana*

Exhale as you go into a deep fold, bringing your nose if possible to your knees. You may try to holf the toes with your fingers. Go only as far as you can without discomfort.

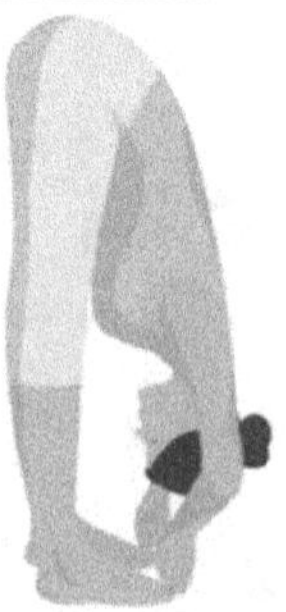

10. **Upward Salute** — *Urdhva Hastasana*

Inhaling straighten your back while your feet are firmly on the groung. Raise your arms from the side and extend the upwards. Let the palms of both hands touch each other while you arch your back and look upwards.

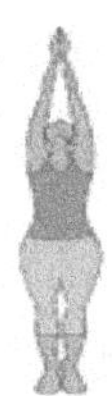

11.**Back to Mountain Pose** — *Tadasana*
Exhale as you come back into Mountain Pose. Bring your hands into prayer position (*Anjali* mudra). Rest your thumbs on your sternum with the fingers pointing up. Repeat the sequence as tolerated – ideally five times.

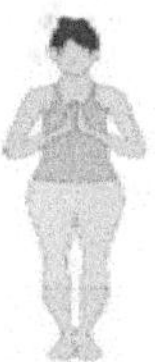

There are several variations of sun salutation but the above is easy to follow with alternating inhalations and exhalations.

As mentioned earlier, the sun salutation sequence burns more calories and is considered a moderate intensity physical work-out. To repeat: physical activity or physical exercise is measured in METs. One MET (Metabolic Equivalent) is approximately equal to a person's resting energy expenditure (e.g. sitting quietly in a chair). Physical activity is categorized into three: light-intensity activities are defined as 1.1 MET to 2.9 METs; moderate-intensity activities are defined as 3.0 to 5.9 METs and vigorous-intensity activities are defined as 6.0 METs or more. Energy expended during sun salutations depends on the intensity of practice. The estimated METs ranges from 2.9 (light intensity) to 7.4 (vigorous). High speed sun salutations therefore meet the criteria for moderate to vigorous exercise, both in adults and children.

SEQUENCE I – 60 POSES

Tadasana

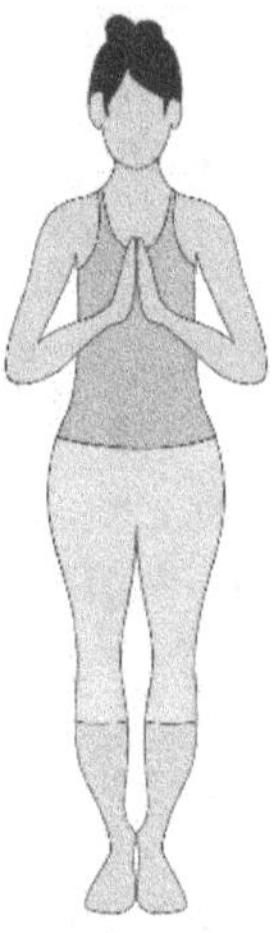

MOUNTAIN POSE
#1

1. **Mountain Pose** (*Tadasana*)

1. Stand upright on your feet. Both feet are close together and pointing straight forward. The weight is spread equally on both feet.
2. The torso/trunk of the body is upright.
3. The eyes are looking straight forward at infinity.
4. The arms are raised, and the hands are brought forward, with the palms opposing each other.
5. The thumbs rest against the breast bone and the fingers point upwards - the prayer position. This is the basic mountain pose with the hands in the prayer pose (*anjali mudra*).

Breathing:

1. Initiation of Pose: Normal breathing
2. Holding Pose: Normal breathing
3. Coming out of pose: Normal breathing

Gaze: Front Infinity

Next Pose: Upward Salute Pose

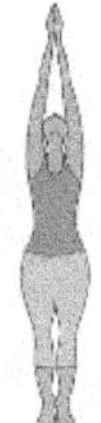

Previous Pose

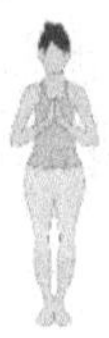

Urdhva Hastasana

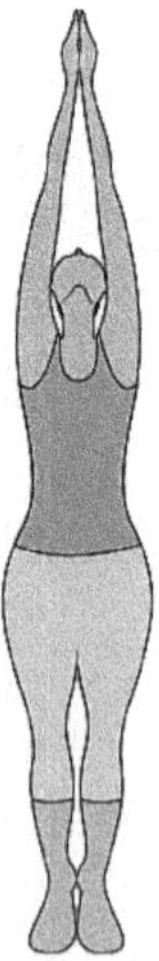

UPWARD SALUTE
#2

2. Upward Salute Pose
(Urdhva Hastasana)

1. Start from the Mountain Pose.
2. Inhaling, stretch your arms above your head and straighten your elbows, keeping the palms touching each other.
3. Still inhaling, raise your body on your toes.
4. Stretch the arms above your head as much as possible, keeping the palms opposed.
5. The arms should touch the ears on each side.
6. The body should be straight and balanced.
7. Breathe normally.
8. Exhaling come out of the pose and go directly into the forward bend pose.

Breathing:

1. Into the pose: inhalation.
2. During the pose: normal breathing.
3. Out of the pose into the next pose: exhalation

Gaze: Sky/ceiling - infinity

Next Pose: Forward Bend

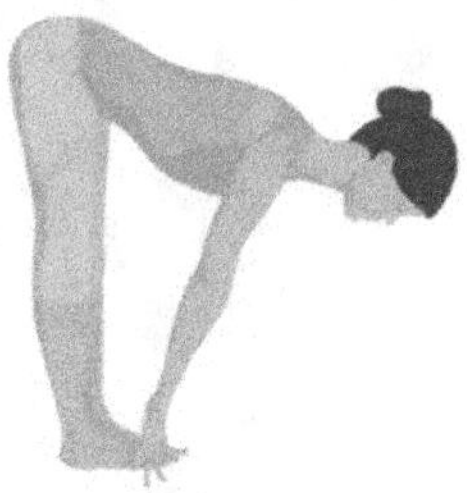

Previous Pose

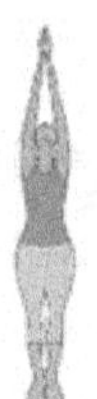

Ardha Uttanasana

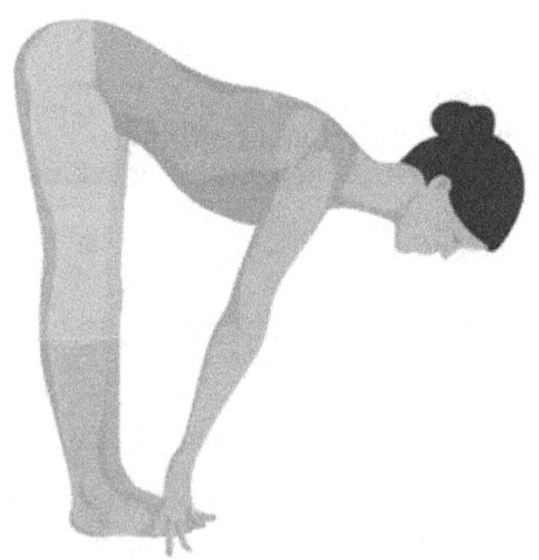

STANDING HALF FORWARD BEND
#3

3. Standing Half Forward Bend
(*Ardha Uttanasana*)

1. From the Mountain Pose, exhaling, bend forward from the waist bringing the chest parallel to the ground.
2. While exhaling, drop your fingers to the corresponding ankles.
3. Lift your head and look forward.
4. Breathe normally.
5. Inhaling, return to the mountain pose.

Breathing:

1. Getting into pose: Exhalation
2. During Pose: Normal breathing
3. Getting out of pose: Inhalation

Gaze: Forward infinity

Transition pose: Mountain Pose

Next Pose: Modified Mountain Pose

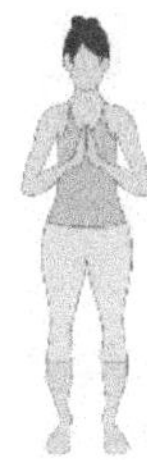

Previous Pose

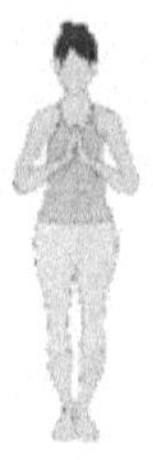

Tadasana – modified

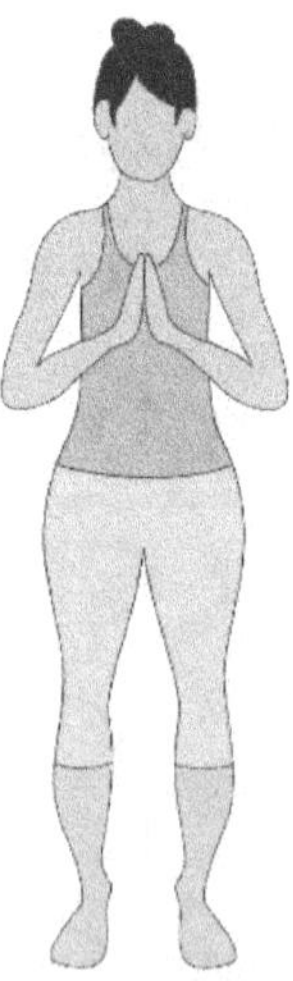

MODIFIED MOUNTAIN POSE
#4

4. Modified Mountain Pose
(Tadasana – modified)

1. Inhaling, spread your feet about hip distance or one foot or so apart.
2. Exhaling, bring your arms down, folded in a prayer position, in front of your chest.
3. The palms should be touching each other softly but firmly and the thumbs against the chest bone.
4. The fingers should be pointing upwards.
5. The feet should be firmly grounded, and the body erect and balanced.
6. Breathe normally.
7. This is also a rest and frequent transition pose.

Breathing:

1. Initiation of Pose: Inhalation/Exhalation
2. Holding of Pose: Normal breathing

Gaze: Front infinity

Next Pose: Crescent Moon in the MMP

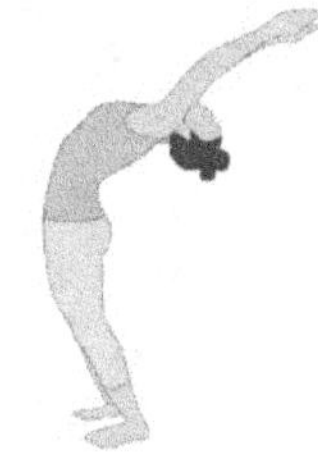

Previous Pose

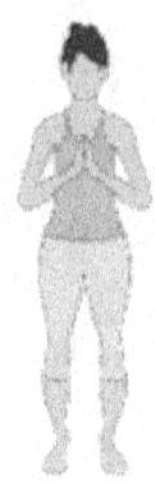

Ardha Chandrasana

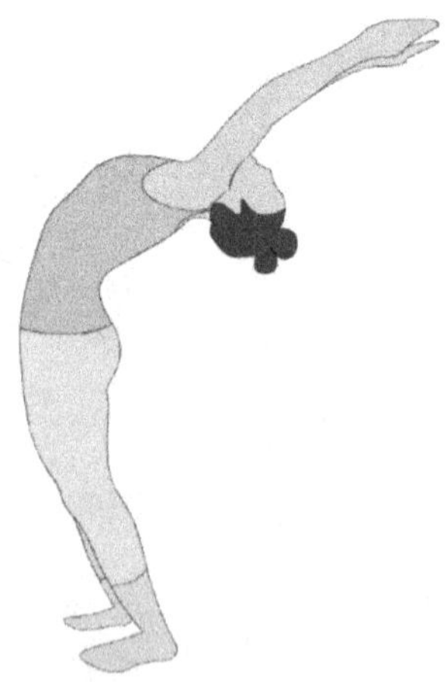

CRESCENT MOON IN MODIFIED MOUNTAIN POSE
#5

5. Crescent Moon
(Ardha Chandrasana)

1. Inhaling from the modified mountain pose, stretch your arms upwards while keeping the palms pressed together.
2. As you continue inhaling, bend your torso backwards and turn your head upwards, facing the sky above.
3. The whole body should be firmly grounded on both feet and arched back like a crescent moon.
4. The knees are not bent.
5. Breathe normally.
6. Exhaling, slowly move to the next pose – deep bend pose.

Breathing:

1. Getting into pose: Inhalation
2. Holding pose: Normal breathing
3. Getting out of pose and into the next pose: Exhalation

Gaze: Upwards sky infinity

Transition pose: None

Next Pose: Deep Forward Bend

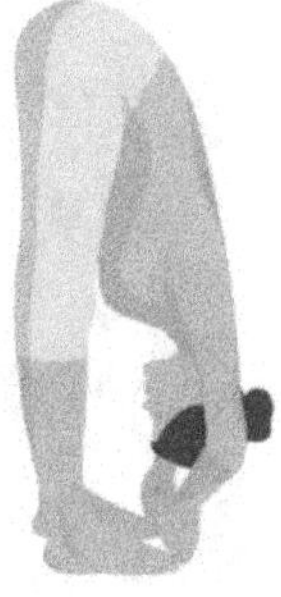

Previous Pose

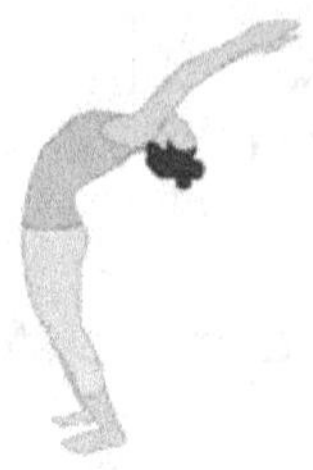

Uttanasana

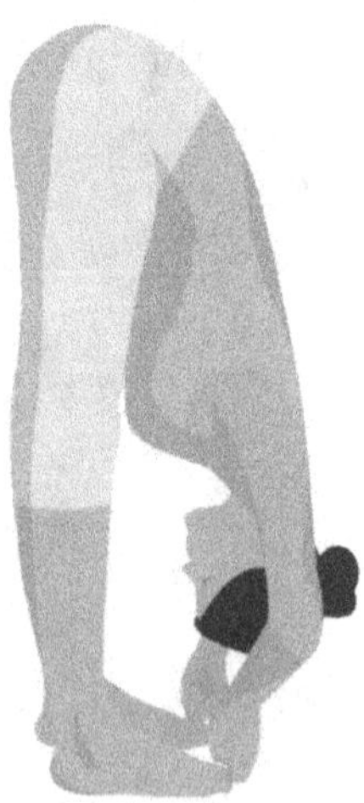

DEEP FORWARD BEND
#6

6. Deep Forward Bend
(Uttanasana)

1. From the crescent moon, instead of going to modified mountain, keep bending forward till your fingers touch your feet.
2. This is done during exhalation in one fluid motion.
3. The feet are firmly on the ground and the knees are kept straight.
4. The body is bent from the hip upwards and folded like a pancake.
5. After the pose is reached, the gaze is tip of the nose.
6. Breathe normally. Gaze is at toes.
7. Inhaling raise the head and upper trunk to an upright position (MMP) and exhaling bring the hands into the prayer position.

Breathing:

1. Getting into pose: exhalation
2. During pose: normal breathing
3. Getting out of pose: inhalation

Gaze: Legs/toes

Transition pose: Modified mountain pose

Next Pose: Forward bend with one leg forward

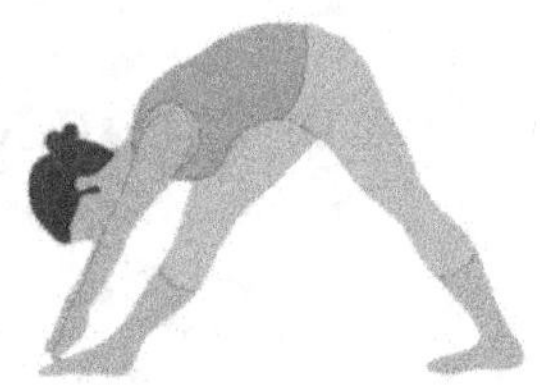

Previous Pose

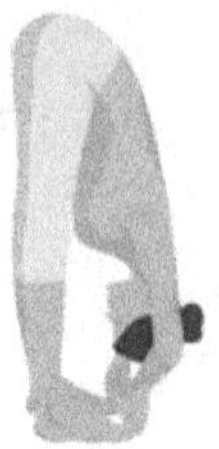

Trikonasana – variation

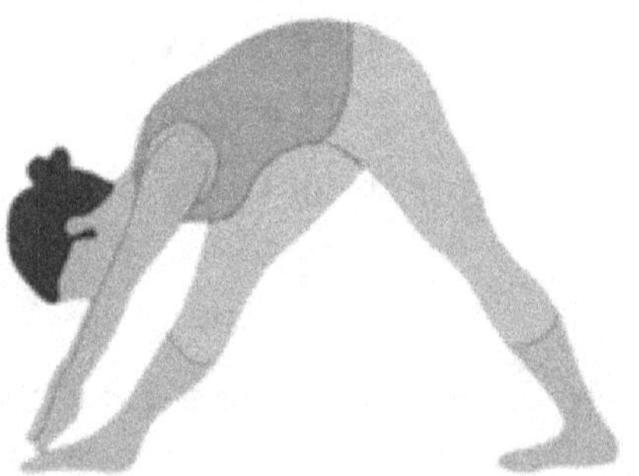

FORWARD BEND RIGHT LEG FORWARD
#7

7. Forward Bend with Right Leg Forward
(Trikonasana – variation)

1. From the modified mountain pose, inhaling, step the right foot forward by about 2-3 feet.
2. The right foot is facing forward and firmly on the ground.
3. At the same time, while inhaling, move your arms upwards over your head.
4. The left foot is turned outwards by about 15 degrees resting firmly on the ground.
5. Exhaling, bend forward from the waist up with the arms gradually bending down towards the extended foot's big toe.
6. Keep both knees extended and both feet firmly on the ground.
7. The gaze is the right big toe.
8. Breathe normally while holding this pose.
9. Inhaling slowly straighten, and exhaling bring your arms back to the prayer position to the modified mountain pose.

Breathing:

1. Getting into the pose: Inhalation/Exhalation
2. During the pose: Normal breathing
3. Getting out of the pose: Inhalation/Exhalation

Gaze: Right big toe

Transition Pose: Modified mountain pose

Next Pose: Forward bend with left leg forward

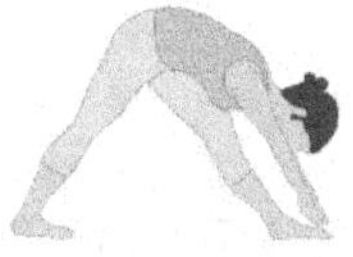

Previous Pose

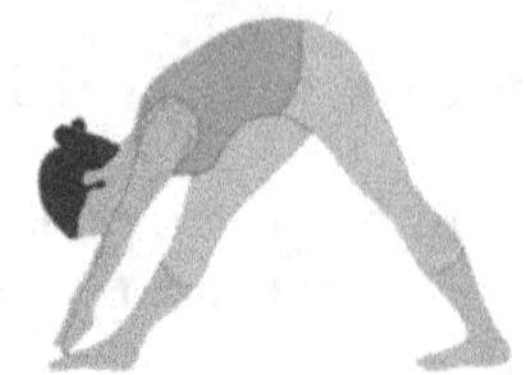

Trikonasana – variation

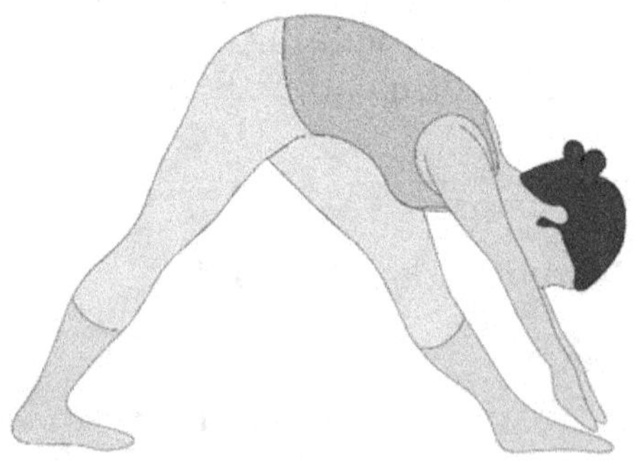

FORWARD BEND LEFT LEG FORWARD
#8

8. **Forward Bend with Left Leg Forward**
(Trikonasana – variation)

1. From the modified mountain pose, inhaling, step the left foot forward 3-4 feet.
2. The left foot is facing forward and firmly on the ground.
3. While continuing to inhale, raise your arms over your head.
4. The right foot is turned outwards by about 15 degrees, resting firmly on the ground.
5. Exhaling, bend forward with both hands towards the left big toe.
6. Both knees are kept straight and both feet firmly on the ground.
7. The gaze is the left big toe.
8. Breathe normally during the hold period.
9. Inhaling, straighten your torso and exhaling bring your arms back to the prayer position to the modified mountain pose.

Breathing:

1. Getting into the pose: Inhalation/Exhalation
2. During the pose: Normal breathing
3. Getting out of the pose: Inhalation/Exhalation

Gaze: Left big toe

Transition pose: Modified mountain

Next pose: Wide legged modified mountain pose

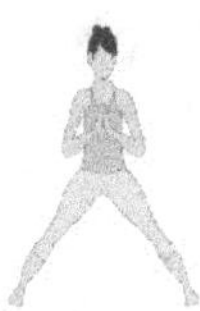

Previous Pose

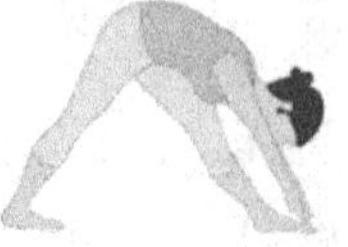

Utthita Tadasana

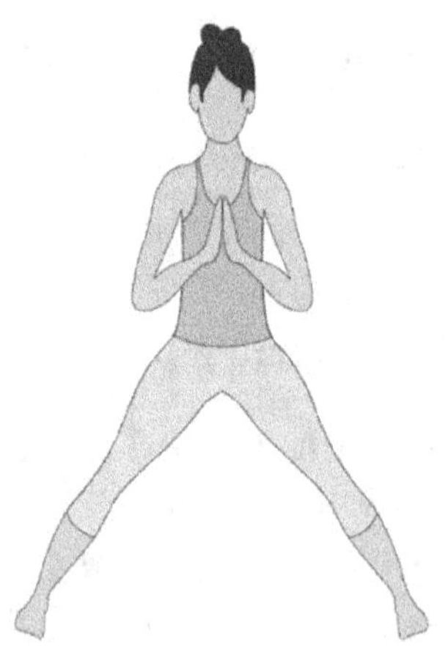

WIDE LEGGED MOUNTAIN POSE
#9

9. **Wide Legged Modified Mountain Pose**
(WLMP) *(Utthita Tadasana)*

1. Start in the modified mountain pose.
2. Inhaling, spread your legs wide apart - 3 to 4 feet apart.
3. Keep your knees straight.
4. Both feet should remain firmly on the ground.
5. Keep your body erect and both arms/hands in the prayer position.
6. Breathe normally

Breathing:

1. Getting into pose: Inhalation
2. During pose: Normal breathing

Gaze: Front infinity

This is also a frequent transition pose.

Next Pose: Wide legged right big toe pose

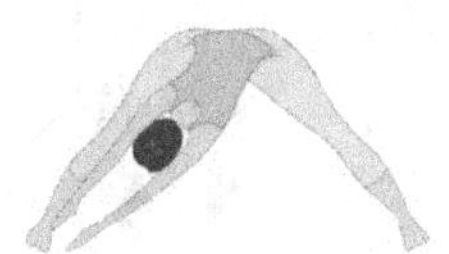

Previous Pose

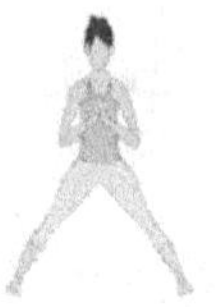

Utthita Trikonsana

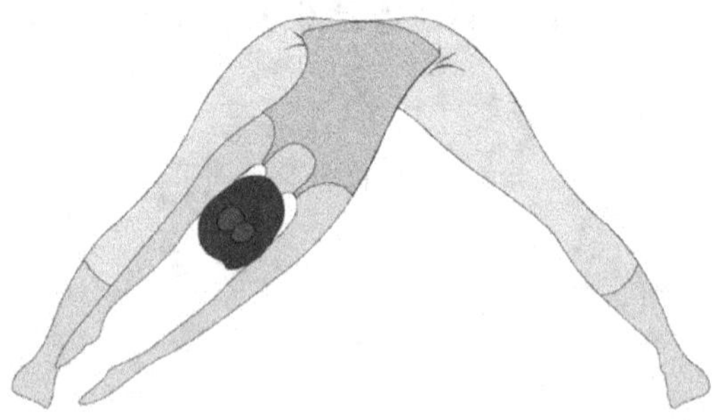

WIDE LEGGED RIGHT BIG TOE POSE
#10

10. **Both Hands to Right Big Toe Pose**
(Utthita Trikonsanas)

1. From the wide legged modified mountain pose,
2. Inhaling, raise both arms towards on the sides (spread out)
3. The elbows are straight, and the arms form a single line parallel to the ground.
4. Exhaling, bend from the torso to the left.
5. At the same time, curve the both arms downwards and to the right reaching over the right ankle and down towards the right big toe – resting the finger tips on the right big toe.
7. Both feet stay firmly on the ground and both knees are kept straight.
8. Breathe normally during the hold.
9 Lift up the right arm and go up with your gaze on the right hand.
10. Bring down the right arm with the hand on the right big toe again.
11. Lift up the left arm up with the gaze following the left hand.
12. Bring down the left arm with the hand on the right big toe again.
13. Inhaling, gradually come back to the upright position with the arms stretched on the sides and exhaling, return to the prayer position in wide legged mountain pose.

Breathing:
1. Getting into the pose: Inhalation/Exhalation
2. During the pose: normal breathing
3. Right arm up: inhalation
4. Right arm down: exhalation
5. Left arm up: inhalation
6. Left arm down: exhalation
7. Getting out of the pose: Inhalation/Exhalation

Gaze: Big toe/thumb of the arm up

Transition pose: Wide legged modified mountain pose

Next pose: Both hands to left big toe pose

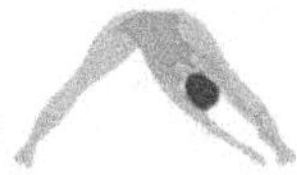

Previous Pose

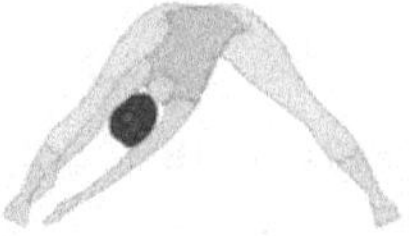

Utthita Trikonsanas

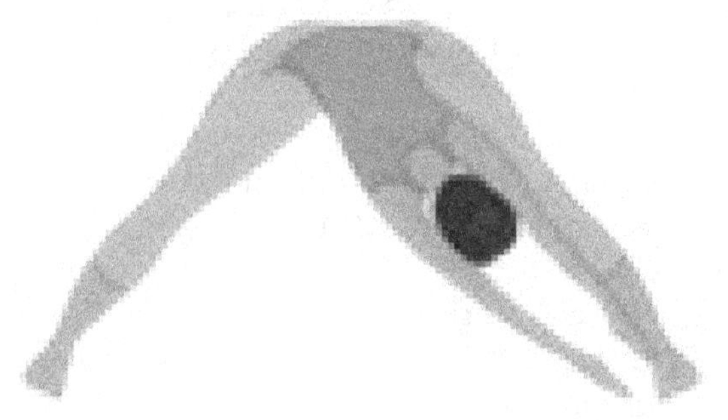

WIDE LEGGED LEFT BIG TOE POSE
#11

11. **Both Hands to Left Big Toe Pose** *(Utthita Trikonsanas)*
1. Start in the wide legged modified mountain pose.
2. Inhaling, raise both arms on the sides.
3. The elbows are straight, and the arms form a single line parallel to the ground.
4. Exhaling, bend from the torso to the left.
6. Curve the both arms downwards and to the left reaching over the left ankle and down towards the left big toe – resting the finger tips on the left big toe.
7. Both feet stay firmly on the ground and both knees are kept straight. Breathe normally during the hold.
8. Lift up the left arm and go up and left with your gaze following the left hand.
9. Bring down the left arm with the hand back on the left big toe again.
10. Lift up the right arm up and towards the right with the gaze following the right hand.
11. Bring down the right arm - hand on the left big toe again.
12. Inhaling, gradually come back to the upright position with the arms stretched on the sides and exhaling, return to the prayer position in wide legged mountain pose.

Breathing:
1. Getting into the pose: Inhalation/Exhalation
2. During the pose: normal breathing
3. Left arm up: inhalation
4. Left arm down: exhalation
5. Right arm up: inhalation
6. Right arm down: exhalation
7. Getting out of the pose: Inhalation/Exhalation

Gaze: Big toe/thumb of the arm up

Transition pose: Wide legged modified mountain pose

Next pose: Crescent moon in wide legged mountain pose

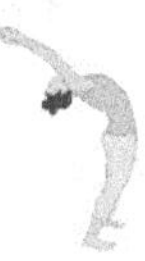

Previous Pose

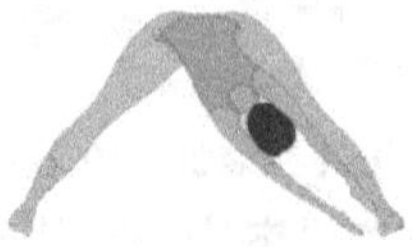

Ardha Chandrasana

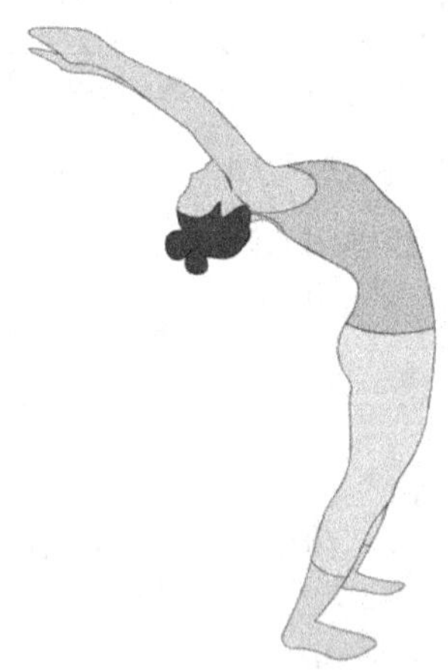

CRESCENT MOON IN WIDE LEGGED MOUNTAIN POSE
#12

12. **Crescent Moon in Wide Legged Mountain Pose**
(Ardha Chandrasana)

1. From the prayer position in the wide legged mountain pose, raise both arms up and backwards, with your body bent backwards concave down. The hands do not touch each other, and the arms are parallel to each other.
2. Hold this pose and breathe normally.
3. Exhaling move gently forward to the next pose.

Breathing:

1. Bending backwards: inhaling
2. In pose: normal breathing. Gaze upwards.
3. Going to next pose: exhaling

Gaze: upwards infinity

Transition pose: None – move smoothly into the next pose

Next pose: Forward bend with palms on floor

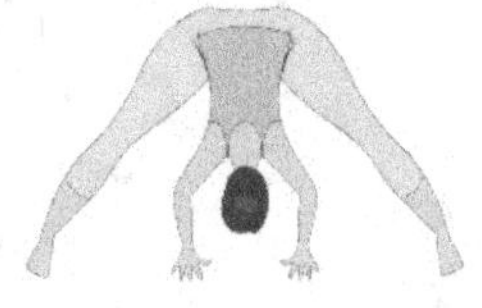

Previous Pose

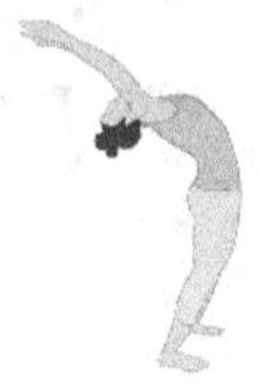

Prasarita Padotansasana

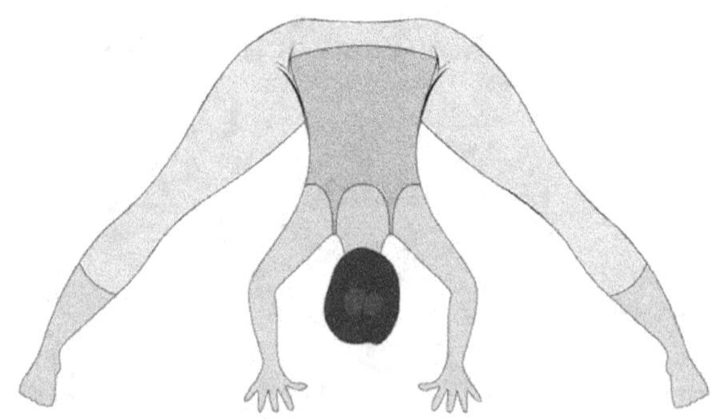

FORWARD BEND WITH PALMS ON FLOOR
#13

13. Forward Bend with Palms on Floor
(Prasarita Padotansasana)

1. From the wide legged mountain pose crescent position, continuously bend forward and put both hands in the middle of both feet as much as possible in line with the feet with the palms on the floor.
2. Breathe normally while holding this position.
3. Inhaling, return to the arms over the head position.
4. Exhaling, return to the prayer position.

Breathing:

1. Bending forward: Exhalation
2. Holding pose: normal breathing
3. Returning to arms above head: inhalation
4. Returning to prayer position in wide legged mountain pose: Exhalation

Gaze: Both hands on floor

Transition pose: Wide legged modified mountain pose

Next pose: Side bend in wide legged mountain pose

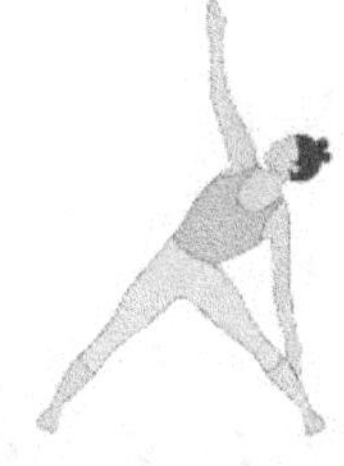

Previous Pose

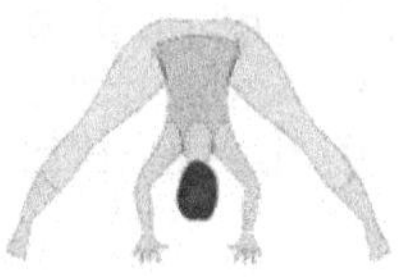

Utthita Parsvakonasana

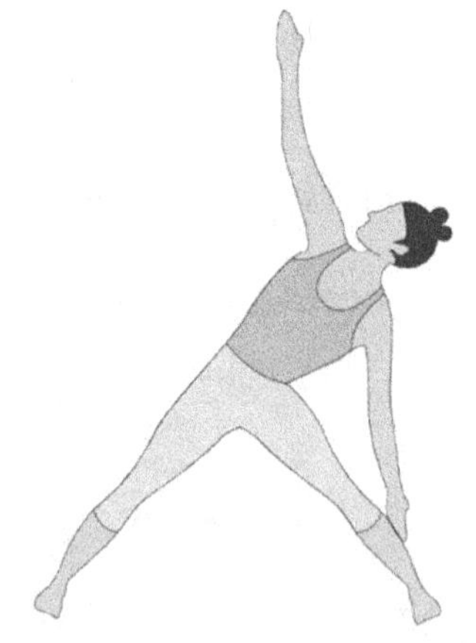

SIDE BEND IN WIDE LEGGED MOUNTAIN POSE LEFT SIDE
#14

14. **Side Bend in Wide Legged Mountain Pose: Left Side**
(Utthita Parsvakonasana)

1. From the wide legged mountain pose turn your left toes facing left. The right foot remains firm with the toes facing forward. Both heels should be aligned along the same line. Look straight forward.
2. Inhaling spread out your arms to the sides at shoulder level.
3. Exhaling, bend at your waist towards the left, and slide your left hand down along the shin of the left leg to the left ankle.
4. The right arm should be simultaneously raised upwards with the shoulders being aligned on top of each other.
5. Your gaze should be upwards at the right-hand thumb.
6. Hold the pose and breathe normally.
7. Inhaling, move back to the arms stretched pose with the left foot now also facing forward and the legs staying wide legged. You are now facing forward.
8. Exhaling, come back to the prayer position.

Breathing:

1. Inhalation while spreading arms.
2. Exhalation on bending.
3. Inhalation on returning.

Gaze: Forward, right thumb during pose, forward

Transition pose: Wide legged mountain pose with prayer hands

Next pose: (R) Side Bend in Wide Legged Mountain Pose

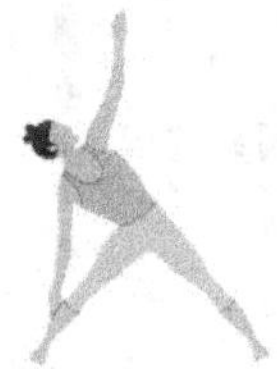

Previous Pose

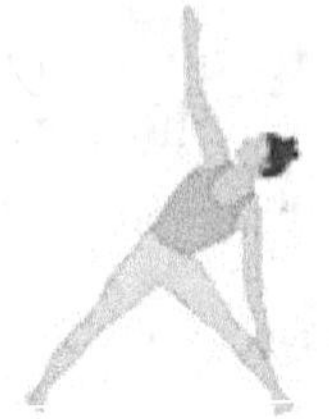

Utthita Parsvakonasana

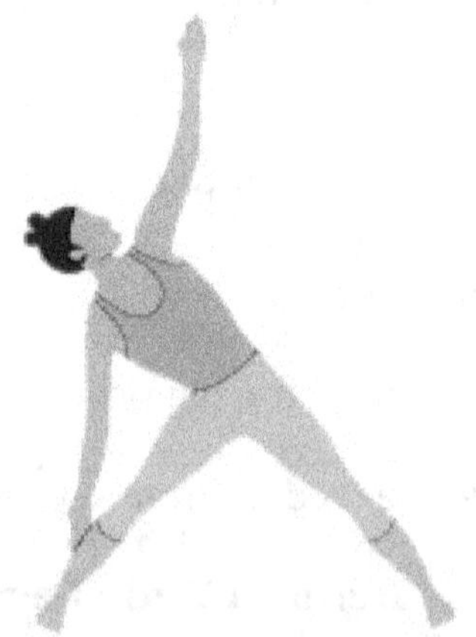

SIDE BEND IN WIDE LEGGED MOUNTAIN POSE RIGHT SIDE
#15

15. Side Bend in Wide Legged Mountain Pose: Right Side *(Utthita Parsvakonasana)*

1. From the wide legged mountain pose turn your right toes facing right. The left foot remains firm with the toes facing forward. Both heels should be aligned along the same line. Look straight forward.
2. Inhaling spread out your arms to the sides at shoulder level.
3. Exhaling, bend at your waist towards the right, and slide your right hand down along the shin of the right leg to the right ankle.
4. The left arm should be simultaneously raised upwards with the shoulders being aligned on top of each other.
5. Your gaze should be upwards at the left-hand thumb.
6. Hold the pose and breathe normally.
7. Inhaling, move back to the arms stretched pose with the right foot now also facing forward and the legs staying wide legged. You are now facing forward.
8. Exhaling, come back to the prayer position.

Breathing:

1. Inhalation while spreading arms.
2. Exhalation on bending.
3. Inhalation on returning.

Gaze: Forward, left thumb during pose, forward

Transition pose: Wide legged mountain pose

Next pose: Warrior I: Right foot forward

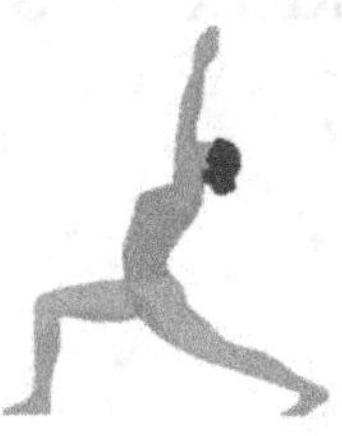

Previous Pose

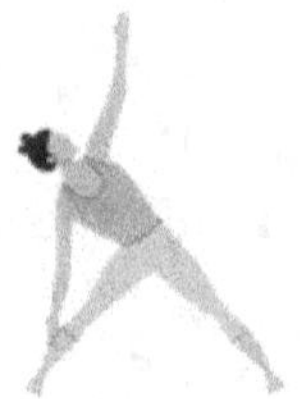

Virabhadrasana I

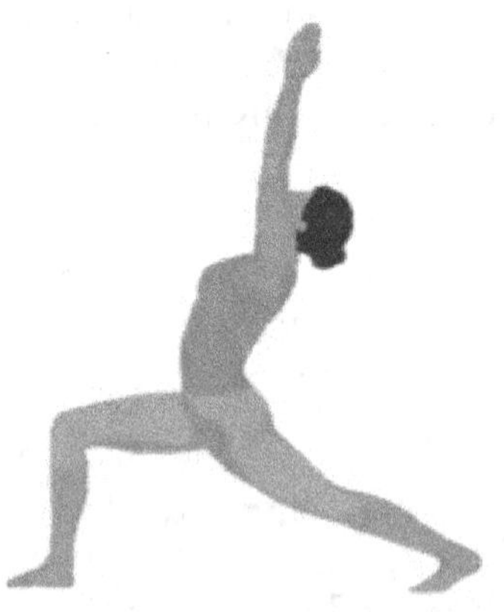

WARRIOR I RIGHT FOOT FORWARD
#16

16. Warrior I: Right Foot Forward - Right Knee Bent
(Virabhadrasana I)

1. From the wide legged mountain pose, bring yourself to the modified mountain pose.
2. Now step your left leg and foot back, behind you, about 1-2 feet. The left foot will be rotated outwards (towards the left front end of the mat) about 30-45 degrees or more. The right foot stays firmly grounded with the toes pointing forward.
3. Now bend the front knee to a 90 degree, with the knee (right knee) directly over the right ankle. You may stretch the left leg further backwards if needed.
4. Both hips stay aligned with the front edge of the mat.
5. From here, reach up with both arms, stretching your belly chest upwards. Reach out as high as you can. The arms can be parallel to each other or the palms can be flat against each other. The biceps are touching the ears.
6. Lift your head back and gaze at the thumbs. You should feel your shoulder blades pressing inwards.
7. Breathe normal while holding this pose.

Breathing: Inhalation during raising arms

Gaze: Upwards/hands

Transition pose: None

Next pose: Forward high lunge in Warrior I

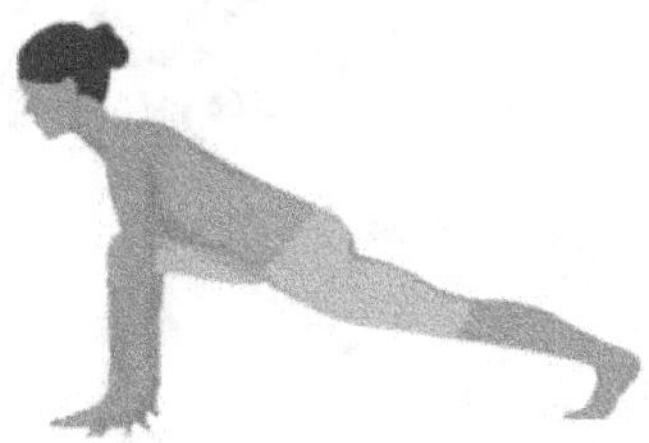

Previous Pose

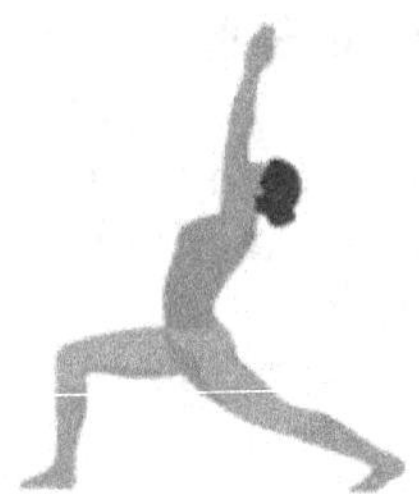

Utthita Ashwa Sanchalanasana

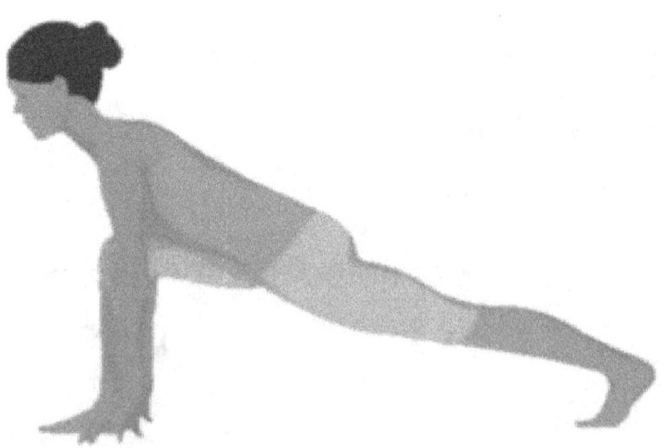

HIGH LUNGE RIGHT KNEE BENT
#17

17. Forward High Lunge in Warrior I Right Foot Forward *(Utthita Ashwa Sanchalanasana)*

1. This pose has no transition – it continues from Warrior I
2. Exhaling bring your arms forward and bend from the waist forward. Let the hands touch the toes or either side of the right ankle – or flat on the ground on either side of the foot.
3. The right knee stays bent at 90 degrees. Your torso will lie on your right thigh.
4. The left leg does not bend and stays straight and firm. The left foot will become raised on the toes. Look forward.
5. Hold position and breathe normally.

Breathing:

1. Exhalation during forward bend.
2. Inhalation on coming out of pose.

Gaze: Forward/infinity

Transition pose: None

Next pose: Reverse Warrior with Right Foot Forward

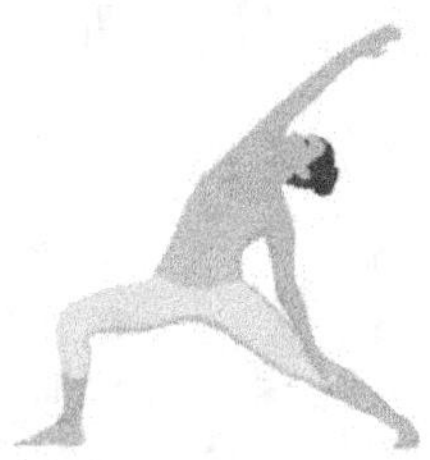

Previous Pose

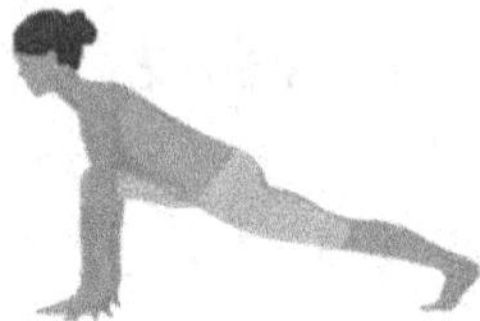

Viparita Virabhadrasana

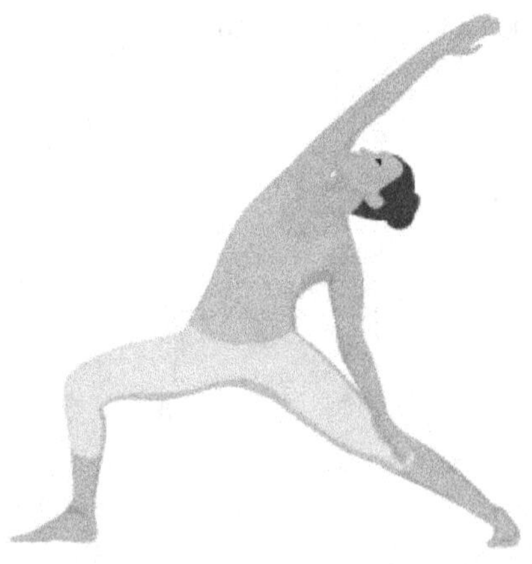

REVERSE WARRIOR I RIGHT KNEE BENT AND FORWARD
#18

18. Reverse Warrior with Right Foot Forward - Right Knee Bent *(Viparita Virabhadrasana)*

1. Start from the forward high lunge pose.
2. Inhaling, lift your torso, arch it backwards and simultaneously raise your right arm towards the ceiling and slide your left arm along the side/back of the left leg. The right bicep muscle should be close to your right ear and your gaze should be on the right thumb.
3. While in this back bend, continue sliding down the left arm on the backside of the left leg. Make sure your right knee stays bent and the right thigh stays parallel to the floor.
4. The waist should be stretched, and the shoulders relaxed.
5. Hold this pose. Breathe normally.
6. Exhaling come back to the wide legged mountain pose in the prayer position.

Breathing:

1. Inhalation during the back stretch.
2. Normal breathing during hold.
3. Exhalation while returning to wide legged Mountain pose.

Gaze: Upwards/infinity

Transition pose: Wide legged mountain pose

Next pose: Warrior I: Left foot forward

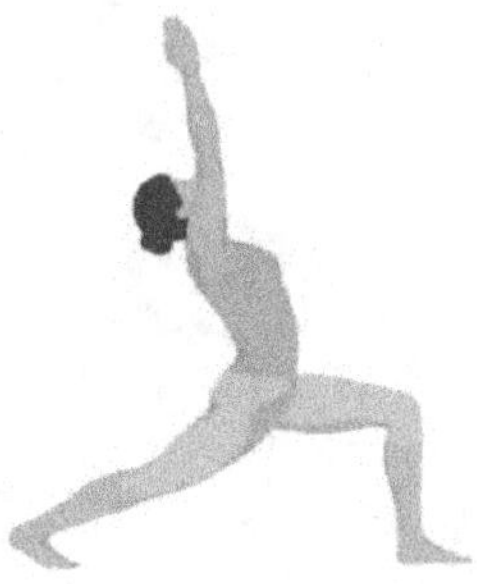

Previous Pose

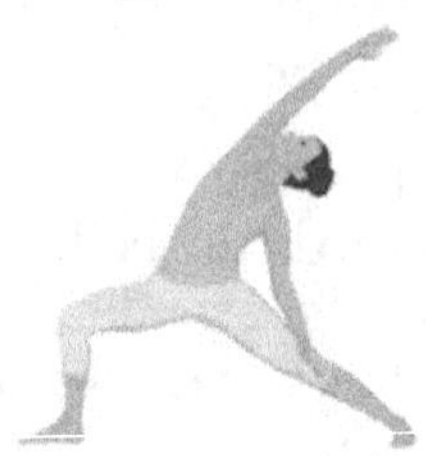

Virabhadrasana I

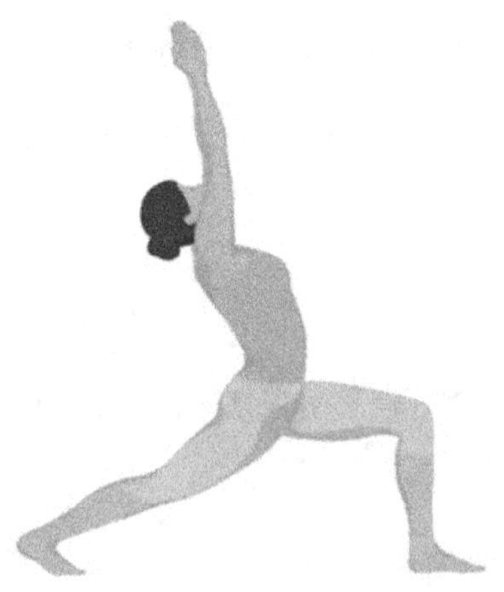

WARRIOR I LEFT FOOT FORWARD
#19

19. Warrior I: Left Foot Forward - Left Knee Bent
(Virabhadrasana I)

1. From the wide legged mountain pose, bring yourself to the modified mountain pose.
2. Now step your right leg and foot back, behind you, about 1-2 feet. The right foot will be rotated outwards (towards the left front end of the mat) about 30-45 degrees or more. The left foot stays firmly grounded with the toes pointing forward.
3. Now bend the front knee (left knee) to a 90 degree, with the knee directly over the left ankle. You may stretch the right leg further backwards if needed.
4. Both hips stay aligned with the front edge of the mat.
5. From here, reach up with both arms, stretching your belly chest upwards. Reach out as high as you can. The arms can be parallel to each other or the palms can be flat against each other. The biceps are touching the ears.
6. Lift your head back and gaze at the thumbs. You should feel your shoulder blades pressing inwards.
7. Breathe normal while holding this pose.

Breathing: Inhalation during raising arms

Gaze: Upwards/hands

Transition pose: None

Next pose: High Lunge Left Foot Forward

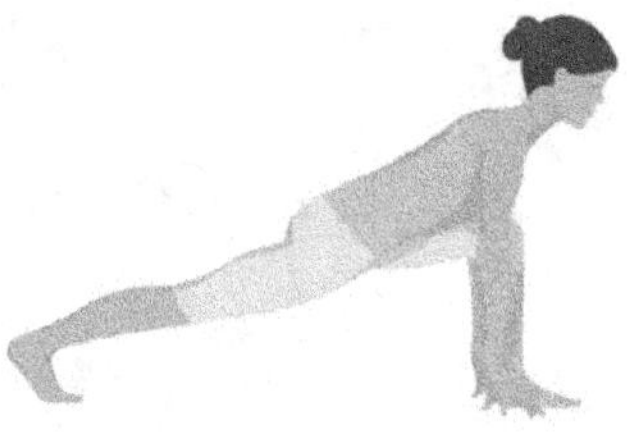

Previous Pose

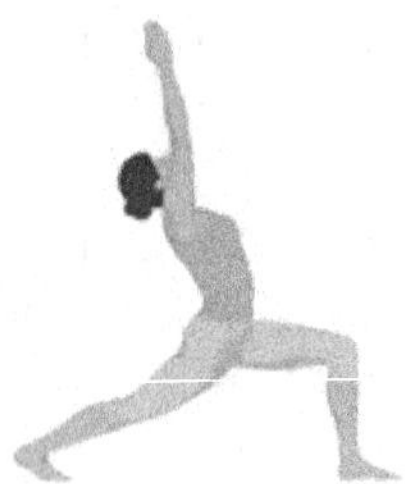

Utthita Ashwa Sanchalanasana

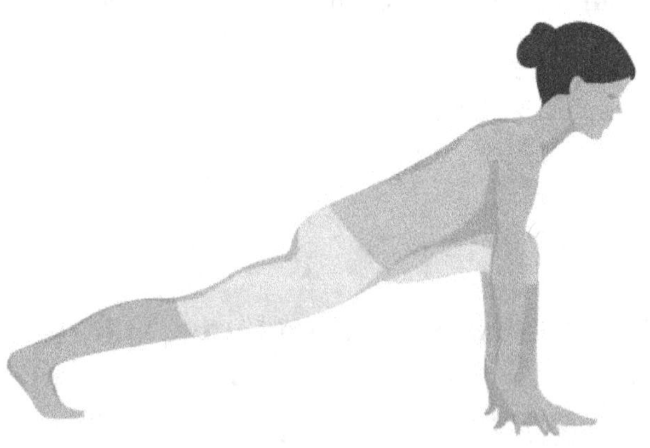

HIGH LUNGE LEFT FOOT FORWARD
#20

20. Forward High Lunge in Warrior I - Left Foot Forward - Left Knee Bent
(Utthita Ashwa Sanchalanasana)

1.   This pose has no transition – it continues from Warrior I
2.   Exhaling bring your arms forward and bend from the waist forward. Let the hands touch the toes or either side of the left ankle – or flat on the ground on either side of the foot.
3.   The left knee stays bent at 90 degrees. Your torso will lie on your right thigh.
4.   The right leg does not bend and stays straight and firm. The right foot will become raised on the toes. Look forward.
5.   Hold position and breathe normally.

Breathing:

1.   Exhalation during forward bend.
2.   Inhalation on coming out of pose.

Gaze: Front/infinity

Transition pose: None

Next pose: Reverse Warrior

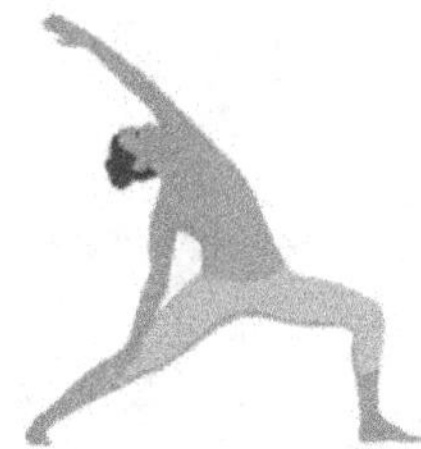

Previous Pose

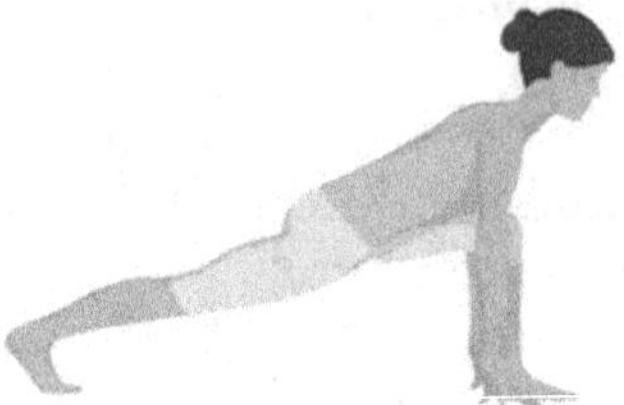

Viparita Virabhadrasana

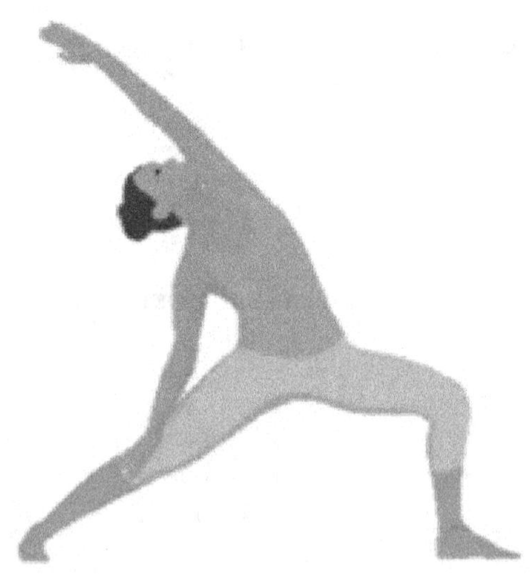

REVERSE WARRIOR I LEFT KNEE BENT AND FORWARD

#21

21. Reverse Warrior with Left Foot Forward
(Viparita Virabhadrasana)

1. This pose has no transition pose
2. Inhaling, lift your torso, arch it backwards and simultaneously raise your left arm towards the ceiling and slide your right arm along the side/back of the right leg. The left bicep muscle should be close to your right ear and your gaze should be on the left thumb.
3. While in this back bend, continue sliding down the right arm on the backside of the right leg. Make sure your left knee stays bent and the left thigh stays parallel to the floor.
4. The waist should be stretched, and the shoulders relaxed.
5. Hold this pose. Breathe normally.
6. Exhaling come back to the wide legged mountain pose in the prayer position.

Breathing:

1. Inhalation during the back stretch.
2. Normal breathing during hold.
3. Exhalation while returning to wide legged Mountain pose.

Gaze: Upwards/infinity

Transition pose: Wide legged mountain pose

Next pose: Warrior II: Right Foot Forward

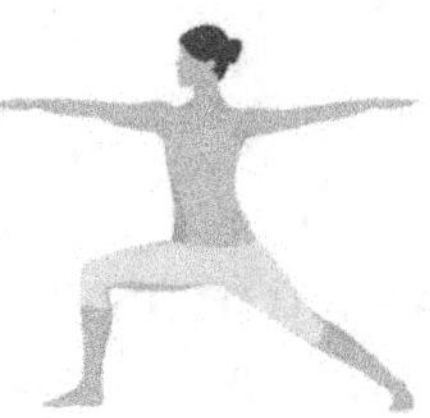

Previous Pose

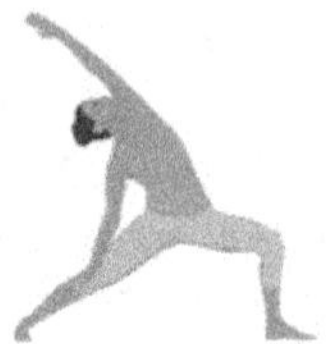

Virabhadrasana II

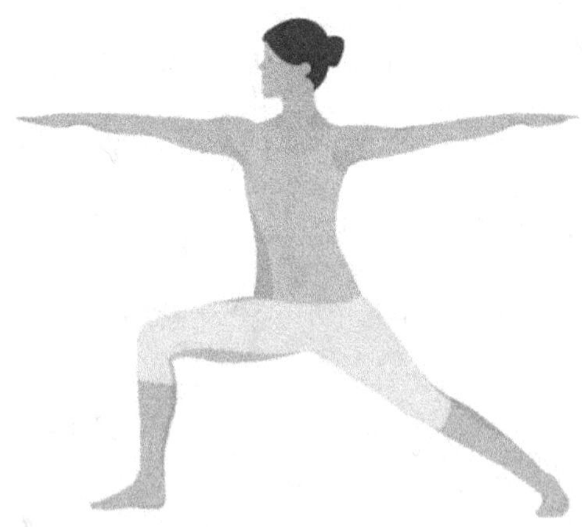

WARRIOR TWO WITH RIGHT LEG FORWARD
#22

22. Warrior II with Right Knee Bent with Twist
(Virabhadrasana II)

1. From the wide legged mountain prayer position, inhaling, spread your arms to the sides, parallel to the floor and in a straight line to each other.
2. Exhaling, turn your right foot 90 degrees to the right and your left foot 45 degrees to the right, and bend the right knee 90 degrees so that the thigh is parallel to the floor.
3. Gaze forward infinity. Hold position. Breathe normally.
4. With your feet firmly planted, exhaling twist your body at the waist to the right, with the arms following the shoulders. The head and gaze follow the rotation.
5. Hold the pose. Breather normally.
6. Inhaling come back to Warrior II.
7. Exhaling turn to the left at the waist with the arms again moving along with the shoulders. The head and gaze follow the rotation.
8. Hold the pose. Breathe normally.
9. Inhaling, come back to Warrior II.
10. Exhaling, bring your feet together in wide legged mountain pose and the arms in prayer pose.

Breathing:

1. Normal during hold.
2. Inhalation during twist and exhalation on return

Transition pose: Wide legged mountain pose

Next pose: Warrior II: Left Foot Forward

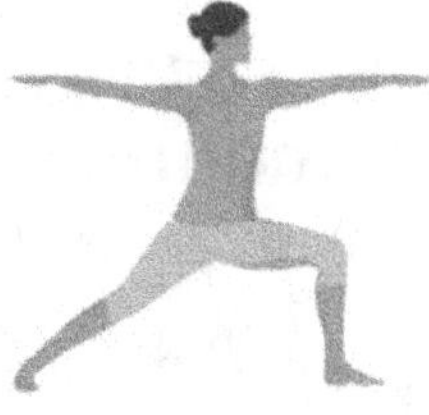

Previous Pose

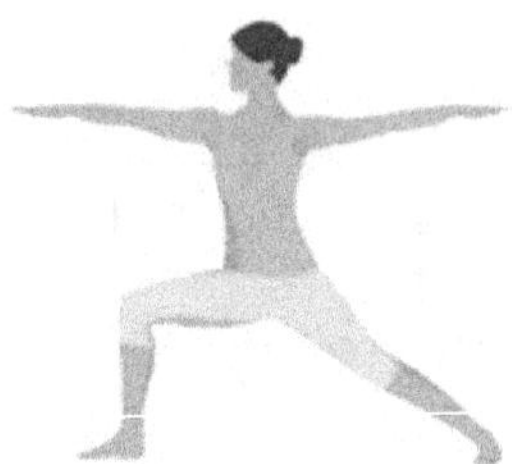

Virabhadrasana II

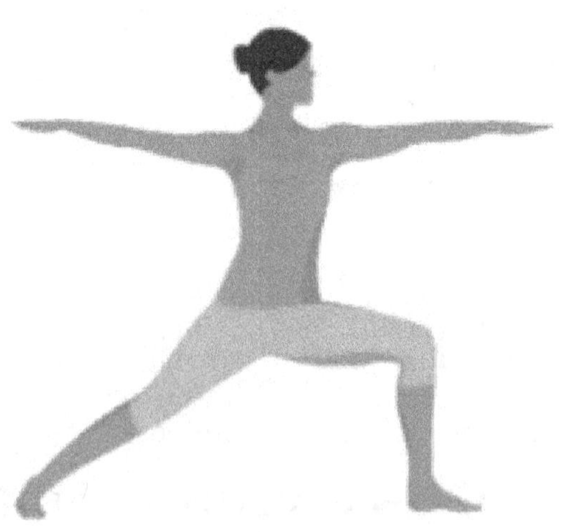

WARRIOR II WITH LEFT LEG FORWARD
#23

23. Warrior II with Left Knee Bent with twist
(Virabhadrasana II)

1. From the wide legged mountain prayer position, inhaling, spread your arms to the sides, parallel to the floor and in a straight line to each other.
2. Exhaling, turn your left foot 90 degrees to the left and your right foot 45 degrees to the left, and bend the left knee 90 degrees so that the thigh is parallel to the floor.
3. Gaze forward infinity. Hold position. Breathe normally.
4. With your feet firmly planted, exhaling twist your body at the waist to the left, with the arms following the shoulders. The head and gaze follow the rotation.
5. Hold the pose. Breather normally.
6. Inhaling come back to Warrior II.
7. Exhaling turn to the right at the waist with the arms again moving along with the shoulders. The head and gaze follow the rotation.
8. Hold the pose. Breathe normally.
9. Inhaling, come back to Warrior II.
10. Exhaling, bring your feet together in modified mountain pose and the arms in prayer pose.

Breathing:

1. Normal during hold.
2. Inhalation during twist and exhalation on returning back

Gaze: Left hand

Transition pose: Modified mountain pose

Next pose: Standing Chair

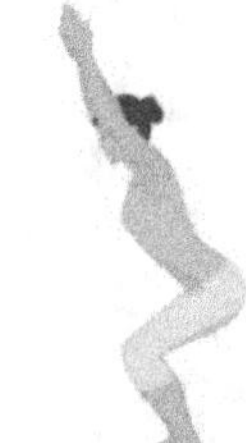

Previous Pose

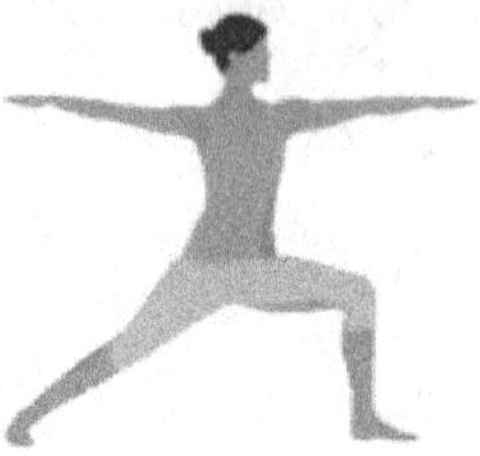

Utkatasana

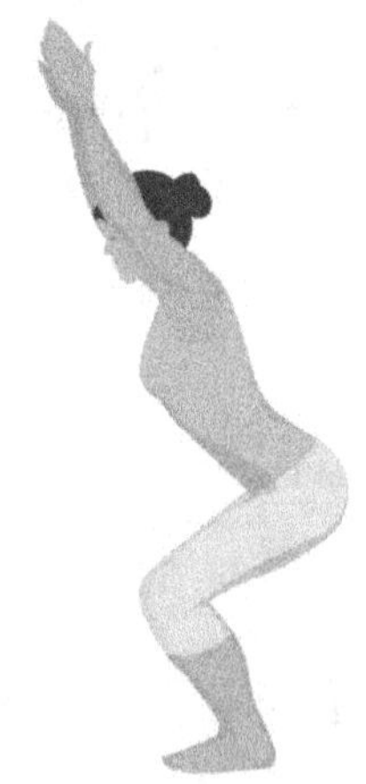

STANDING CHAIR
#24

24. Standing Chair *(Utkatasana)*

1. From the mountain pose, inhale and raise your arms above your head, perpendicular to the floor. They should be parallel to each other with the palms facing inwards.
2. Exhaling, bend your knees to make the thighs as parallel to the floor as possible, without losing balance. The torso should be at right angles to the thighs. The thighs should be parallel to each other. Gaze is front infinity. Breathe normal during this hold.
3. Inhaling, straighten your knees and gently return to the mountain pose with arms in the air above the head.
4. Exhaling, bring the arms back to the prayer position.

Breathing:

1. Exhalation during downward move.
2. Normal during hold.

Gaze: Front/infinity

Transition pose: None

Next pose: Garland Pose

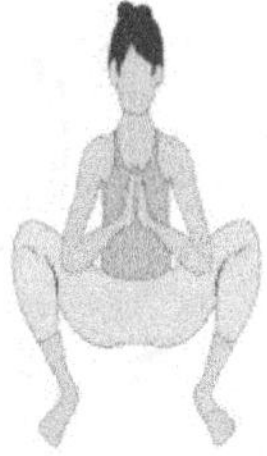

Previous Pose

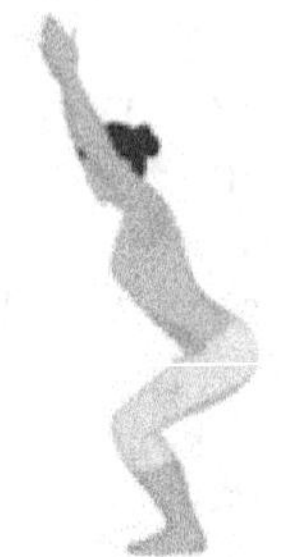

Malasana

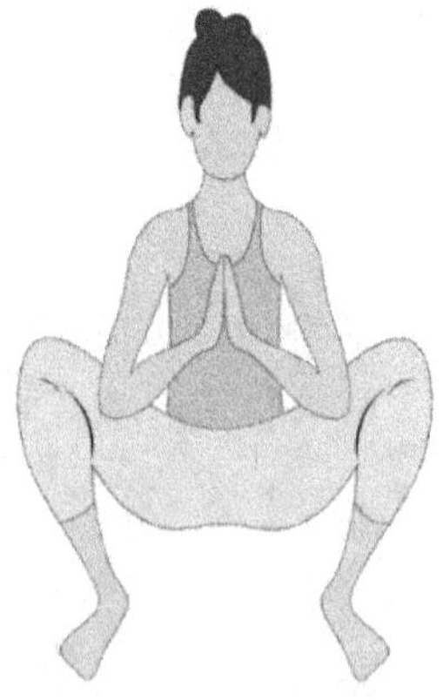

GARLAND POSE
#25

25. Garland Pose *(Malasana)*

1. From the chair position, exhaling, slowly assume a squat pose with the feet flat on the floor. Inhale.
2. Exhaling, bend your torso forward and fit your prayer hands between the thighs with the elbows against the inner side of the knees. Push the knees against the elbows. The palms stay pressed against each other.
3. Hold Pose. Gaze is the finger tips. Breathe normally.

Breathing:

1. Exhalation on way down.
2. Normal during hold.

Gaze: Front/infinity or hands

Transition pose: None

Next pose: Hero Pose

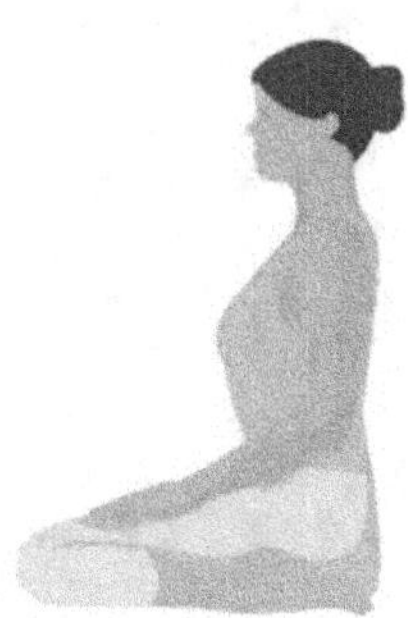

Previous Pose

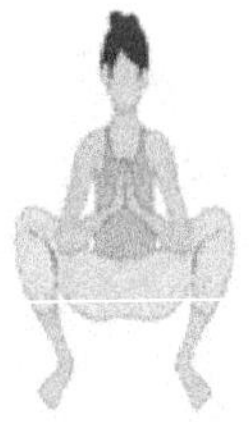

Virasana

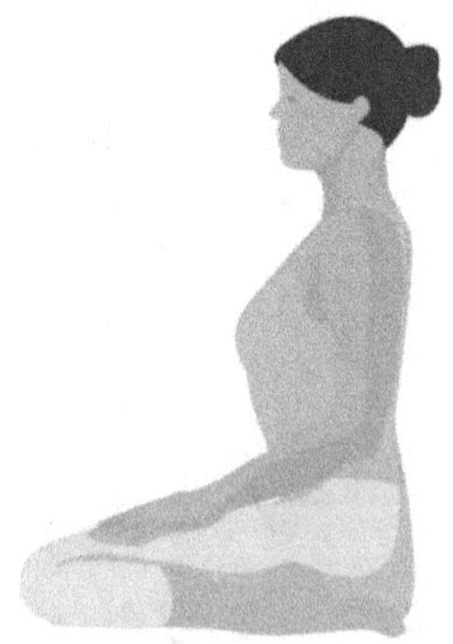

HERO POSE
#26

26. Hero Pose (*Virasana*)

1. From the garland pose, Inhaling, bend forward and place your knees on the floor.
2. Move your calves out with your toes touching the floor. The lower legs are now on the floor,
3. Place your hands on the thighs. Sit in between the two legs. Your position should be snug with the outer thighs in contact with your inner calves.
4. Chest should be straight up with the face looking forward. Gaze would be front infinity.
5. Hold position. Breathe normally. This is also a rest position. If you are unable to sit on the floor, sit on a folded blanket placed in between your thighs/feet.

Breathing: Normal

Gaze: Front infinity

Transition pose: None

Next pose: Easy Pose

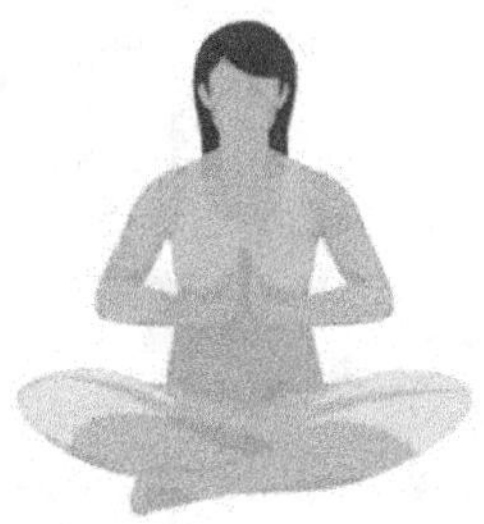

Previous Pose

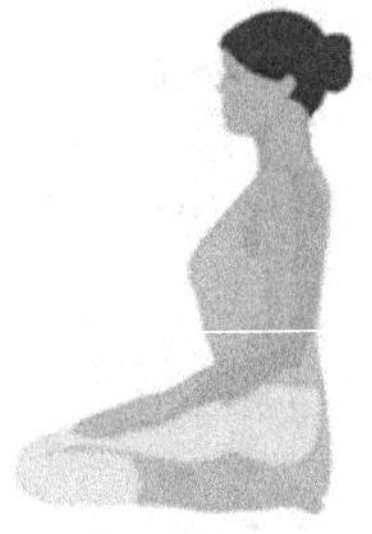

Sukasana

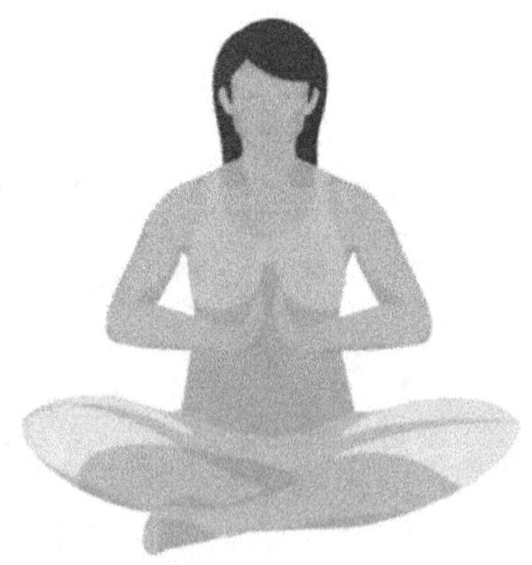

EASY POSE
#27

27. Easy Pose *(Sukhasana)*

1. Breathing normally, place both hands on the floor and straighten out the legs in front of you.
2. Sit up straight. (This is the *dandasana* pose)
3. Cross your legs in front of you and fold them near your torso.
4. With the knees wide apart, tuck your feet beneath the opposite knee. Either shin can be on top – it is good to alternate on different days.
5. Place your palms on the knees, facing down or up, and relaxed.
6. Hold this pose. Gaze is front infinity. Breathe normally. This is also a rest position.

Breathing: Normal

Gaze: Front infinity

Transition pose: None

Next pose: Butterfly Pose

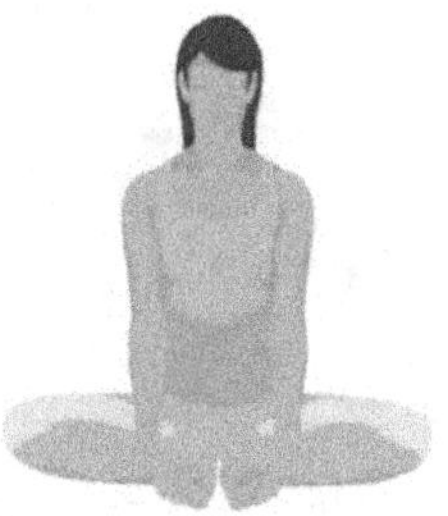

Previous Pose

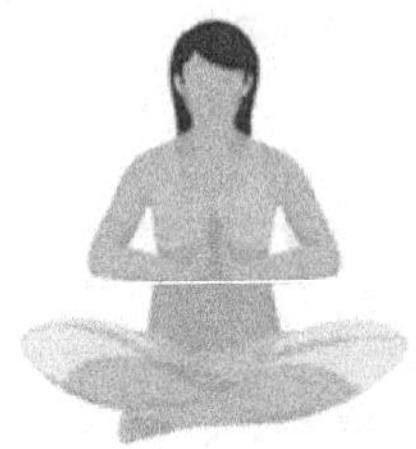

Badhakonasana

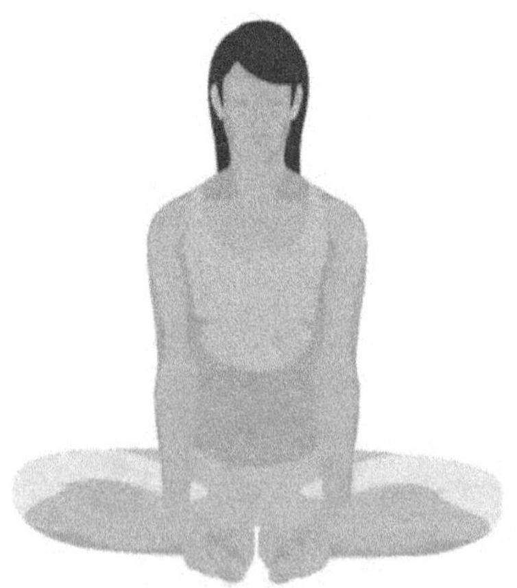

BUTTERFLY POSE
#28

28. Butterfly Pose *(Badhakonasana)*

1. From the easy pose, spread your knees apart and let your soles touch each other.
2. Bending a little forward if you need to, hold both feet firmly with your hands.
3. Pull the heels of the feet towards your groin.
4. Push your knees and thighs against the floor – and start flapping the legs up and down like a butterfly. Your hold on the feet should remain firm and in the same position near the groin. Do ten flaps at a fair pace while breathing normally.
5. Return to the butterfly pose – exhaling, bend your torso forward and touch your head to the feet. Hold for 10 seconds while breathing normally.
6. Inhaling, lift your torso up and return to the initial butterfly pose.
7. From the butterfly pose, let go off the feet and straighten both legs keeping your body perpendicular to them and erect. Hand are on the thighs. This is the *dandasana* pose (staff pose).

Breathing:

1. Normal during flapping.
2. Exhalation during forward bend.
3. Normal during hold.

Gaze: Toes

Transition pose: None

Next pose: *Dandasana* pose (staff pose)

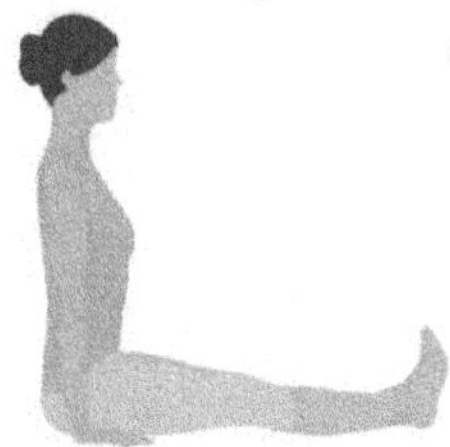

Previous Pose

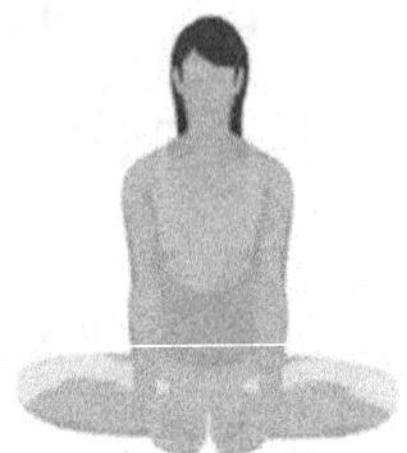

Dandasana

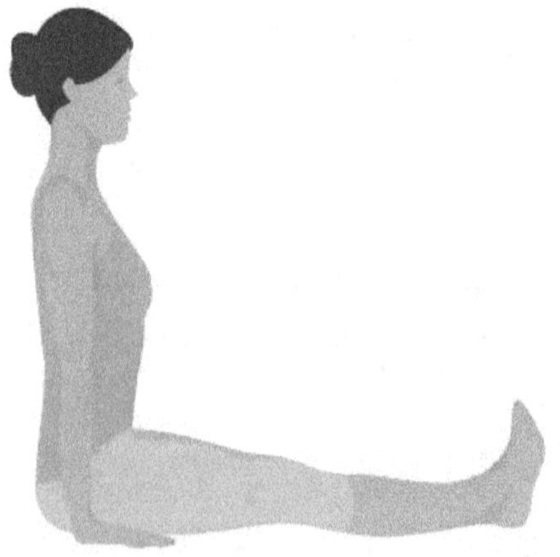

STAFF POSE
#29

29. Staff Pose *(Dandasana)*

1. From the butterfly pose, straighten your legs in front of you.
2. Your thighs and lower legs and heels of the feet are resting on the floor.
3. Keep your back upright.
4. The palms of the hands are brought besides you with the fingers pointing forwards.

Breathing: Normal during hold

Gaze: Toes/front infinity

Transition pose: None

Next pose: Half Bound Forward Bend

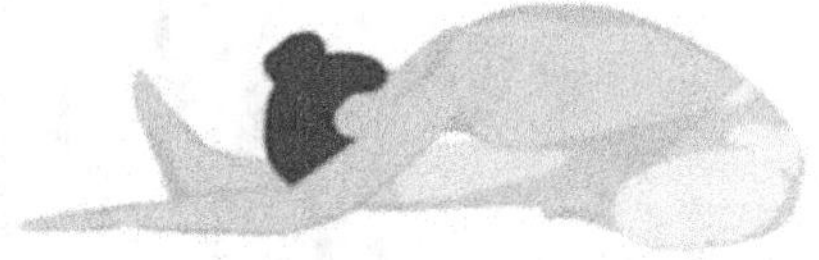

Previous Pose

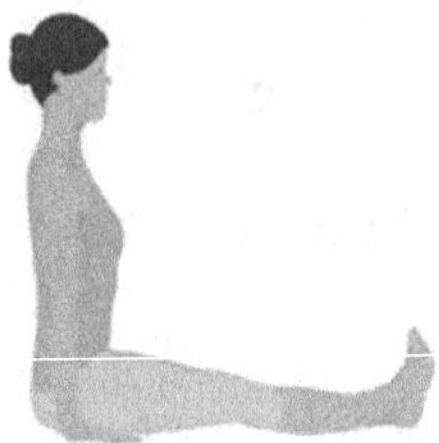

Ardha Baddha Padmottanasana

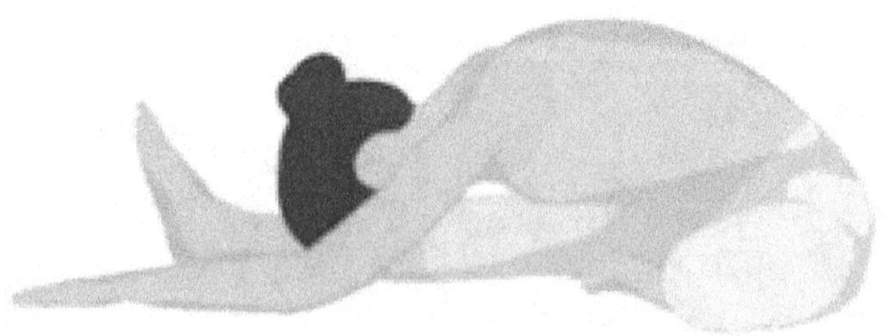

**HALF BOUND FORWARD BEND
RIGHT LEG STRAIGHT**
#30

30. Half Bound Forward Bend - Right Leg Straight
(Ardha Baddha Padmottanasana)

1. Start with the *dandasana* pose.
2. Holding the left knee with the left arm, bend the left knee and holding the left foot with the right hand, pull the foot against the inside of the right leg.
3. The legs stay touching the floor and the right leg is kept straight.
4. Extend both arms towards the right foot and clasp the foot with both hands.
5. Bend the torso forward with the nose touching the right leg – anywhere from the knee downwards. (or as close as you can get)
6. Continue holding the foot with both hands while bent forward. Hold this pose.
7. Breathe normally.
8. Inhaling, get out of the pose to the *dandasana* pose.

Breathing:

1. Exhalation during forward bend.
2. Inhalation on coming out of pose.

Gaze: Toes/knee

Transition pose: *Dandasana* pose

Next pose: Half Bound Forward Bend - Left Leg Straight

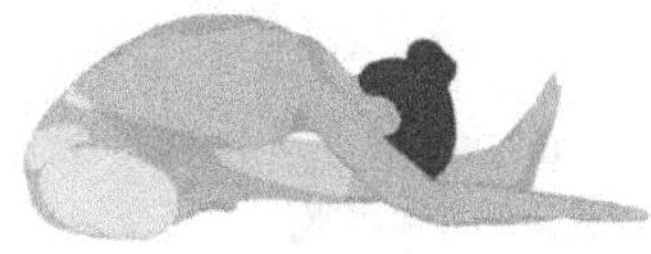

Previous Pose

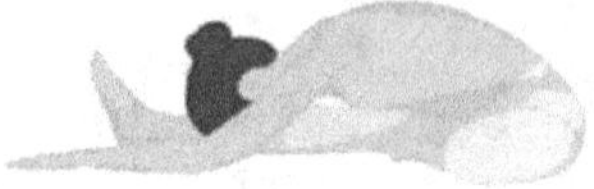

Ardha Baddha Padmottanasana

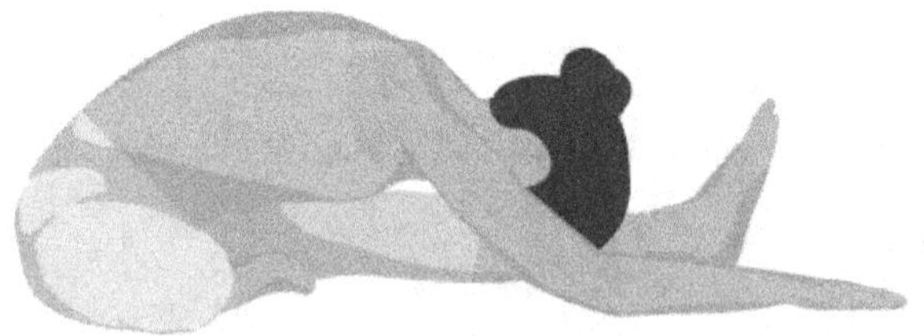

HALF BOUND FORWARD BEND – LEFT LEG STRAIGHT
#31

31. Half Bound Forward Bend - Left Leg Straight
(*Ardha Baddha Padmottanasana*)

1. Start with the *dandasana* pose.
2. Holding the right knee with the right arm, bend the right knee and holding the right foot with the left hand, pull the foot against the inside of the left leg.
3. The legs stay touching the floor and the left leg is kept straight.
4. Extend both arms towards the left foot and clasp the foot with both hands.
5. Bend the torso forward with the nose touching the left leg – anywhere from the knee downwards. (or as close as you can get)
6. Continue holding the foot with both hands while bent forward. Hold this pose.
7. Breathe normally.
8. Inhaling, get out of the pose to the *dandasana* pose.

Breathing:

1. Exhalation during forward bend.
2. Inhalation on coming out of pose.

Gaze: Toes/knee

Transition pose: *Dandasana* pose

Next pose: Thunderbolt

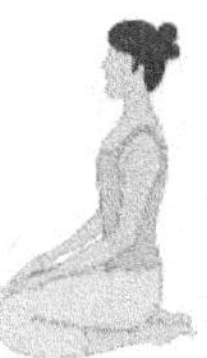

Previous Pose

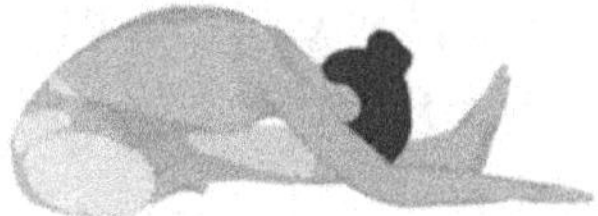

Vajrasana

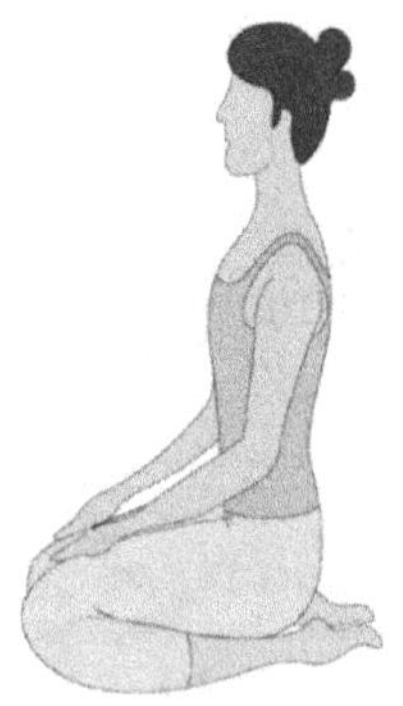

THUNDERBOLT
#32

32. **Thunderbolt** *(Vajrasana)*

1. From the *dandasana* pose, using one hand and palm, lift your body.
2. Bend the knees and slide the legs back.
3. The knees, legs and feet are close together.
4. The soles of the feet are facing upwards.
5. Lower your torso and let your buttocks rest on the heels.
6. Lift and straighten your torso so that it is perpendicular to the floor.
7. The hands rest on the thighs/knees.
8. Gaze is forward.
9. This pose is like the hero pose, except that your bottom is now resting on your thighs and not on the floor between the thighs.

Breathing: Normal during hold

Gaze: Front/infinity

Transition pose: None

Next Pose: Crescent Moon in Thunderbolt Pose

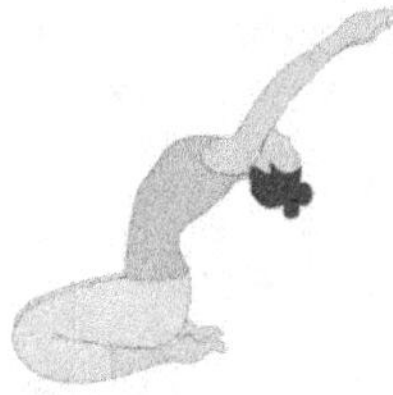

Previous Pose

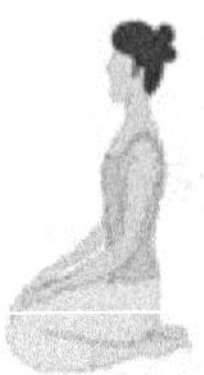

Ardha Chandrasana in Vajrasana pose

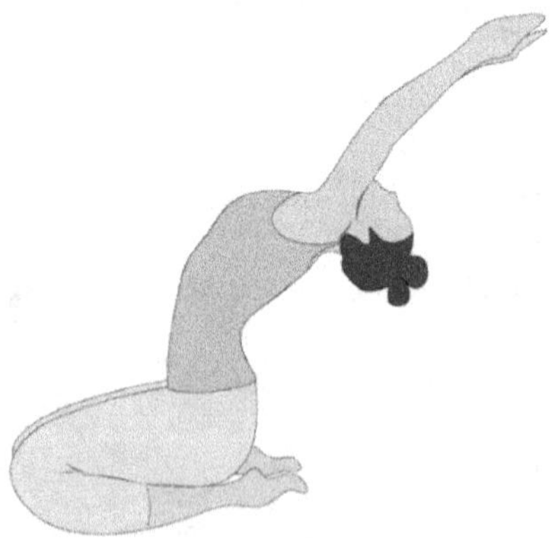

CRESCENT MOON IN THUNDERBOLT POSE
#33

33. Crescent Moon in Thunderbolt Pose
(Ardha Chandrasana in Vajrasana pose)

1. Start in the thunderbolt pose.
2. Inhaling, raise your hands above your head and while bending your torso concave backwards, continue to move your hands to the back.
3. The arms are parallel to each other and the face is looking upwards.
4. The gaze is upwards infinity.
5. Hold this pose and breathe normally.
6. Exhaling, come back to the *vajrasana* position.

Breathing:

1. Inhalation during back bend.
2. Normal breathing during hold.
3. Exhalation on moving upper body forward.

Gaze: Upwards/infinity

Transition pose: None

Next pose: Child Pose

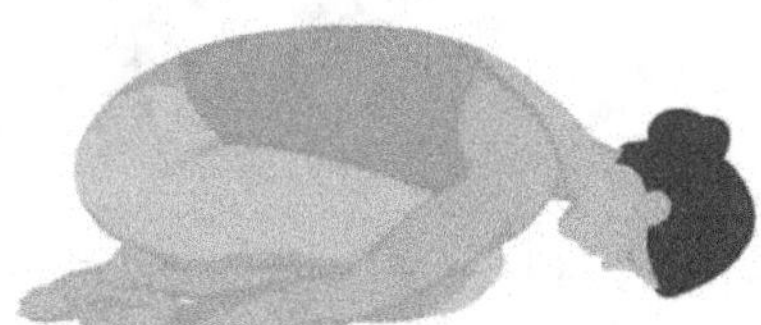

Previous Pose

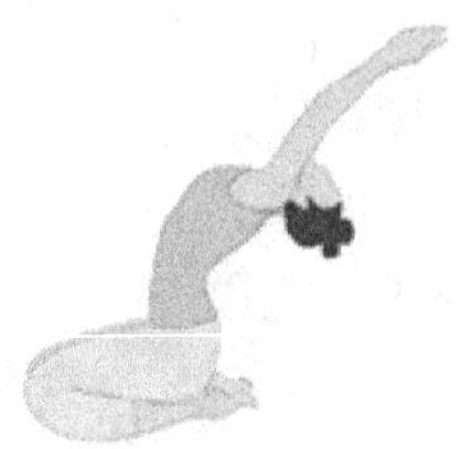

Balasana

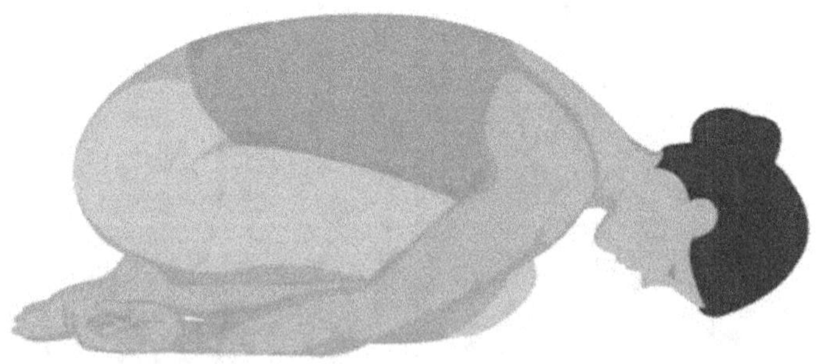

CHILD POSE
#34

34. **Child Pose** (*Balasana*)

1. Start in the thunderbolt crescent moon pose. *(Ardha Chandrasana in Vajrasana pose)*
2. Exhaling, bend your torso forward, with your chest resting on your thighs and your forehead touching the floor.
3. Your arms at the same time move backwards with the palms facing up. The arms should be straight and extended with the palms resting on the floor or clasped behind your buttocks.
4. The buttocks should continue to rest on your heels.
5. The forehead continues to touch the floor with the eyes closed.
6. Hold this position. Breathe normally.
7. Inhaling, move back to Thunderbolt pose.

Breathing:

1. Exhalation getting into pose.
2. Normal breathing during hold.
3. Inhalation on moving to next pose.

Gaze: Knees

Transition pose: None

Next pose: Extended puppy pose

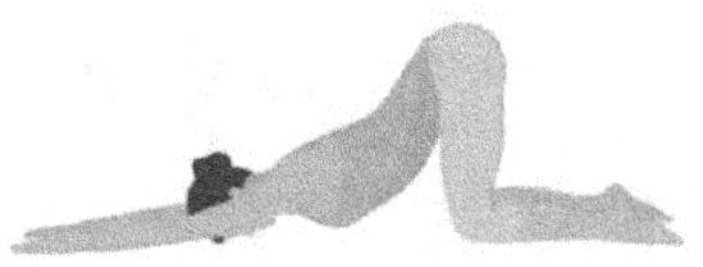

Previous Pose

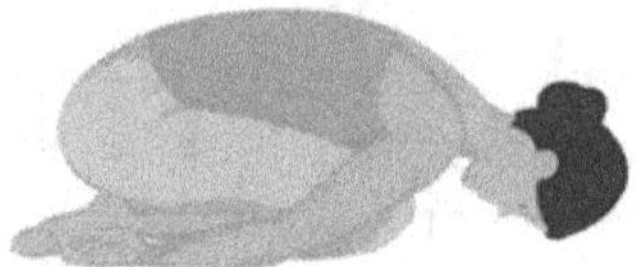

Uttana Shishosana

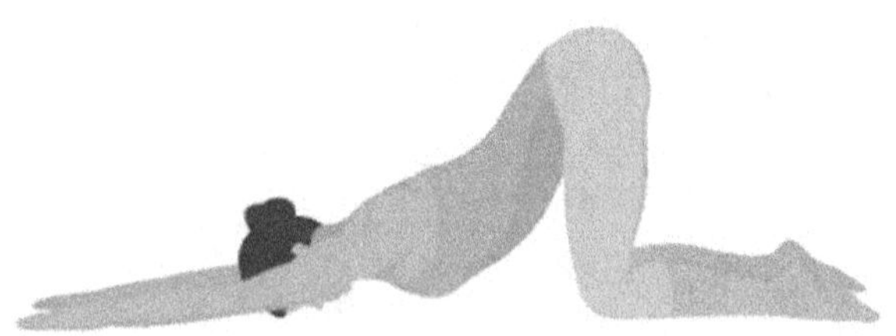

EXTENDED PUPPY POSE
#35

35. **Extended Puppy Pose** *(Uttana Shishosana)*

1. Exhaling, bend your torso forward and placing your palms on the floor in front of you, slowly slide them forward till your thighs are off your legs and perpendicular to the legs.
2. Face is downwards, and you stretch forward as much as you can with the thigh and legs in a constant position.
3. Hold this pose and breathe normally.
4. Inhaling, get back into the Thunderbolt pose

Breathing:

1. Exhalation during forward bend.
2. Normal during hold.
3. Inhalation during return to Thunderbolt pose.

Gaze: Floor

Transition pose: *Vajrasana*

Next pose: Standing Thunderbolt Pose

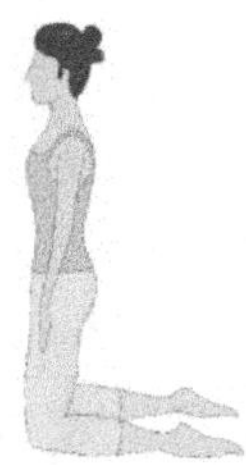

Previous Pose

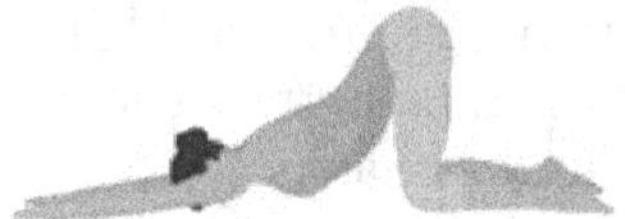

(Modified - Standing) *Vajrasana*

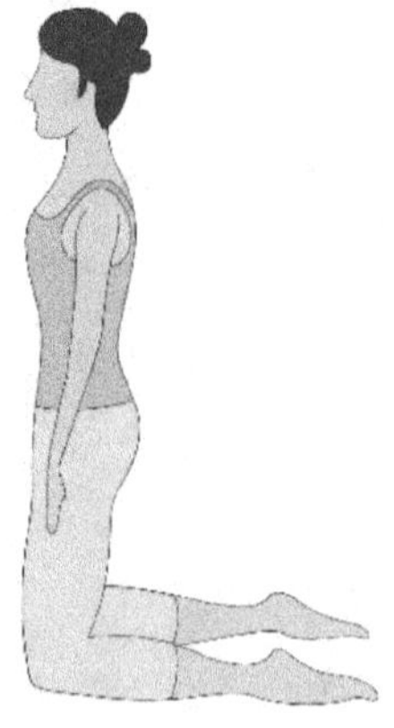

STANDING THUNDERBOLT POSE
#36

36. Standing Thunderbolt Pose
(Modified Vajrasana)

1. From the *vajrasana* position, raise your torso from the knees so that the thighs are perpendicular to the lower legs. Your torso is straight and upright.
2. The arms are by the side with the fingers facing downwards.

Breathing:

1. Inhalation while moving the torso up.
2. Normal breathing while holding the pose.

Gaze: Front/Infinity

Transition pose: None

Next Pose: Gate latch – right leg extended

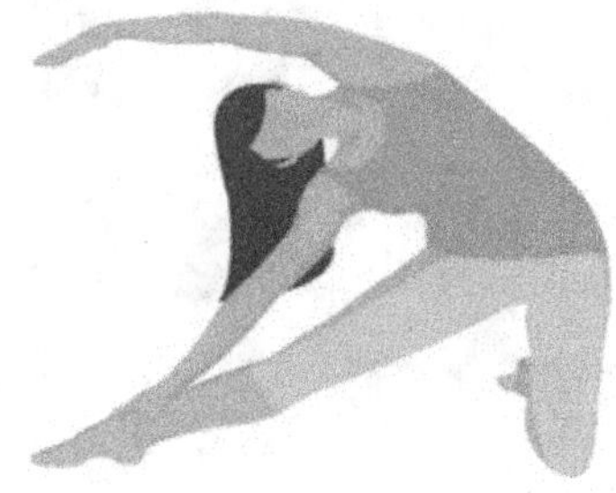

Previous Pose

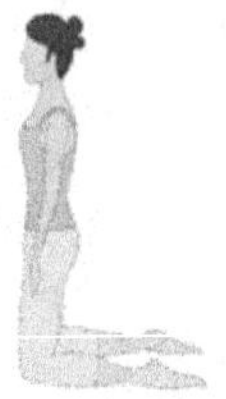

Parighasana

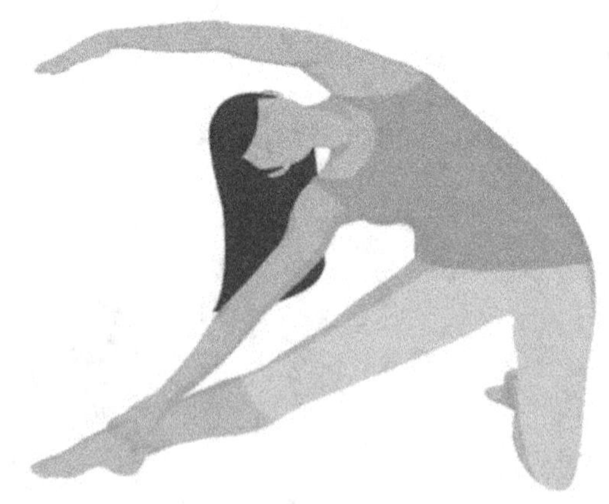

GATE LATCH POSE RIGHT LEG EXTENDED
#37

37. **Gate Latch: Right Leg Extended** *(Parighasana)*

1. From the standing *vajrasana* position, extend your right leg towards the right in line with your body – perpendicular to the left thigh. The knee cap should be facing the ceiling and the toes stretched to the right.
2. Extend both arms out with palms facing down.
3. Inhaling, extend your arms out at shoulder height to the sides to shoulder-height with your palms facing down.
4. Slowly slide your right arm along the right thigh down the shin and to the ankle. At the same time extend your left arm and hand towards the ceiling, with the left biceps resting against your left ear. The left fingers are facing upwards now, as is your gaze.
5. Rest your right hand along your left thigh, shin, or ankle. Turn your left palm upward, and reach your left arm to the left, so your bicep rests against your left ear. The head will be pushed to the right. Turn your gaze up toward the ceiling.
6. Face forwards infinity. Hold and breathe normally.
7. Release the pose and come back to the standing thunderbolt position.

Gaze: Front/infinity

Transition Pose: Standing thunderbolt

Next Pose: Gate latch – left leg extended

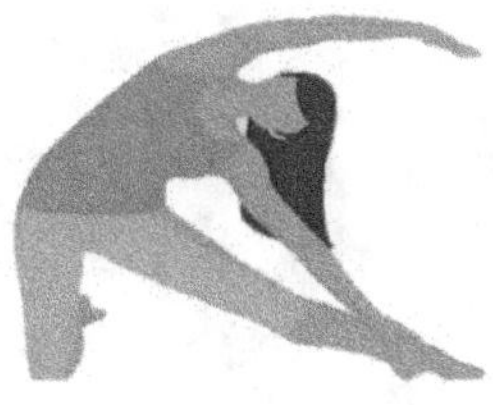

Previous Pose

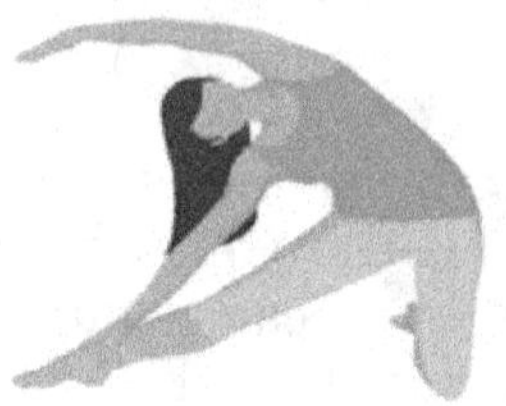

Parighasana

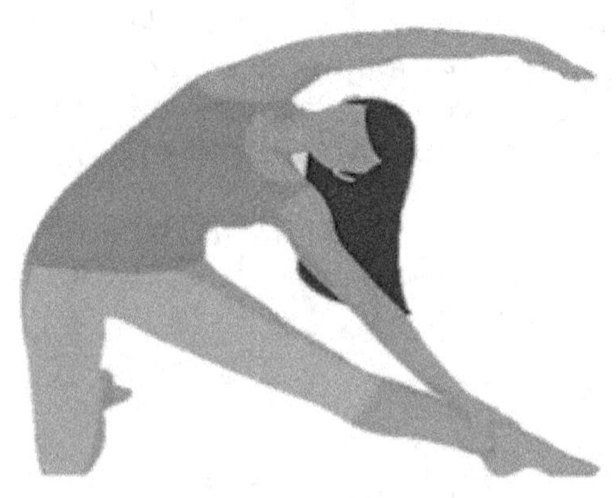

GATE LATCH LEFT LEG EXTENDED
#38

38. Gate Latch: Left Leg Extended *(Parighasana)*

1. From the standing thunderbolt position, extend your left leg towards the left in line with your body – perpendicular to the right thigh. The knee cap should be facing the ceiling and the toes stretched to the left.
2. Extend both arms out with palms facing down.
3. Inhaling, extend your arms out at shoulder height to the sides to shoulder-height with your palms facing down.
4. Slowly slide your left arm along the left thigh down the shin and to the ankle. At the same time extend your right arm and hand towards the ceiling, with the right biceps resting against your right ear. The right fingers are facing upwards now, as is your gaze.
5. Rest your left hand along your left thigh, shin, or ankle. Turn your right palm upward, and reach your right arm to the left, so your bicep rests against your left ear. The head will be pushed to the left. Turn your gaze up toward the ceiling.
6. Face forwards infinity. Hold and breathe normally.
7. Release the pose and come back to the Staff position.

Gaze: Front/infinity

Transition Pose: Standing thunderbolt

Next Pose: Downward Facing Dog

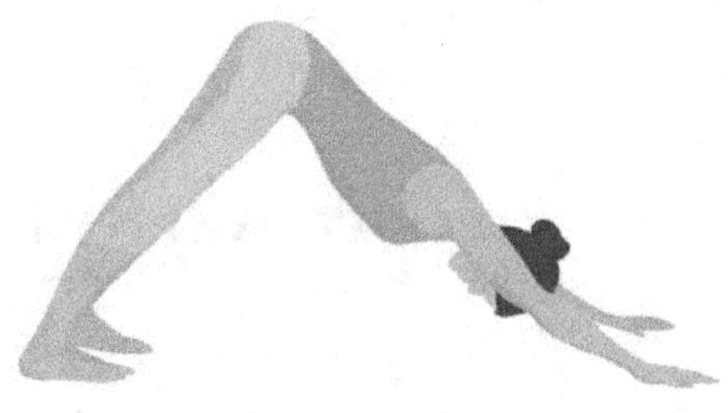

Previous Pose

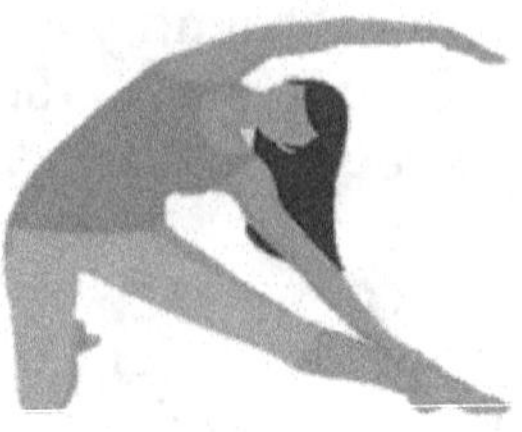

Adho Mukha Svanasana

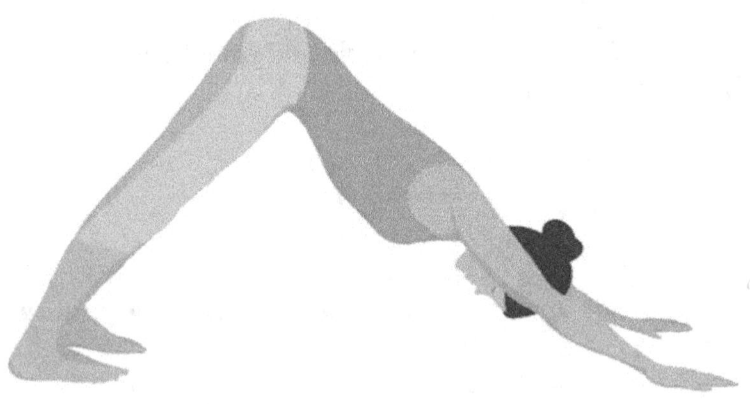

DOWNWARD FACING DOG
#39

39. Downward Facing Dog *(Adho Mukha Svanasana)*

1. From the thunderbolt position, bend forward and put your palms, shoulder length apart, on the floor in front of you.
2. Spread the fingers and have the weight of the front body rest on the palm and fingers.
3. Now gradually lift your knees off the floor, straightening your legs and having the soles of the feet flat on the ground.
4. The pelvis is now raised, and you are in an inverted 'V' shape.
5. The face is looking down.
6. The muscles in the arms and legs should be tight and firm.
7. Hold this pose.

Breathing: Normal breathing during hold

Gaze: Forward hands/floor/back legs

Transition Pose: None

Next Pose: Low Lunge with right knee bent

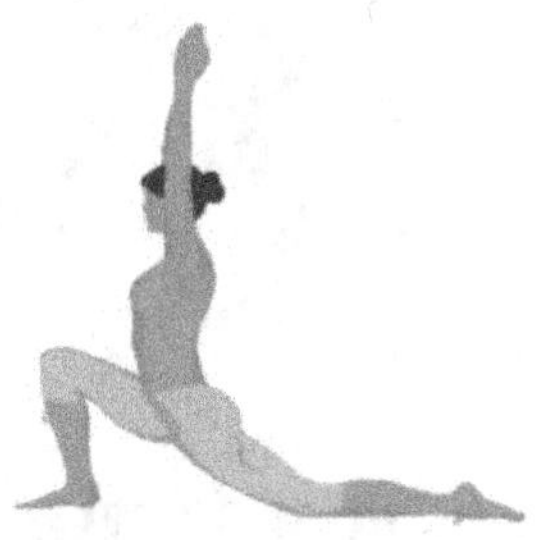

Previous Pose

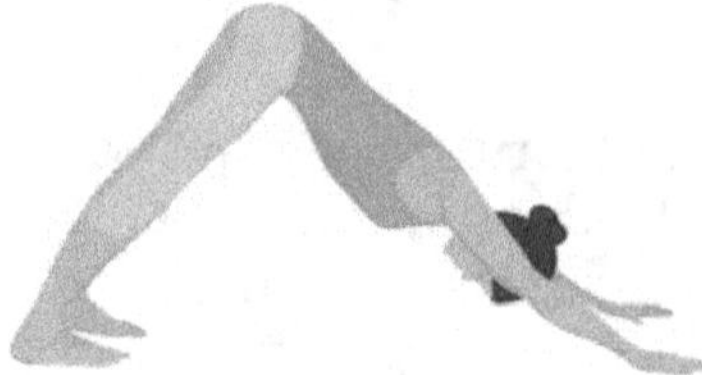

Anjaneyasana

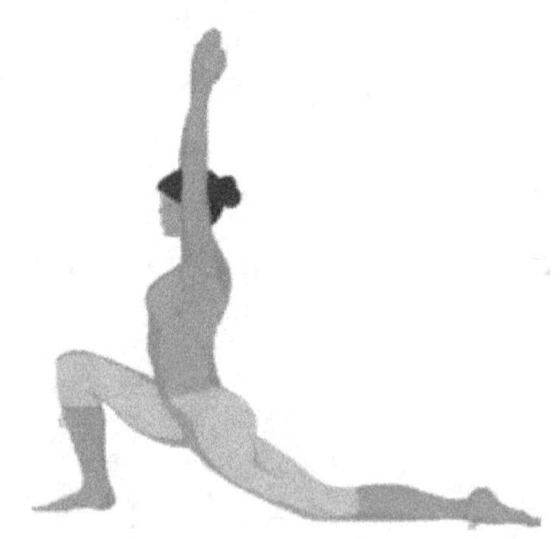

LOW LUNGE RIGHT KNEE BENT
#40

40. Low Lunge: Lizard: Right Knee Front and Bent *(Anjaneyasana)*

1. Start in the downward dog pose.
2. Exhaling, step your right foot forward between your hands, with the sole flat on the floor.
3. The right knee is above the right ankle/heel.
4. Now lower your left knee towards the floor, so that the left knee and the left lower leg is now on the floor.
5. The left foot is sole upwards on the floor.
6. Slide backwards with the left leg if needed to get into a comfortable stretch – the right knee stays at 90 degrees bent position.
7. Now slowly raise both arms upwards so that they are perpendicular to the floor.
8. The biceps are touching both ears and the finger tips are pointing upwards.
9. Face forwards infinity. Hold this pose.
10. Slowly bring your hands down and put your palms on the floor besides the right knee.
11. Pushing your palms downwards, slowly stretch your right leg backwards and slowly raising your torso, come into the downward facing dog pose.

Gaze: Front Infinity

Transition Pose: Downward Dog

Next pose: Low lunge – left knee bent

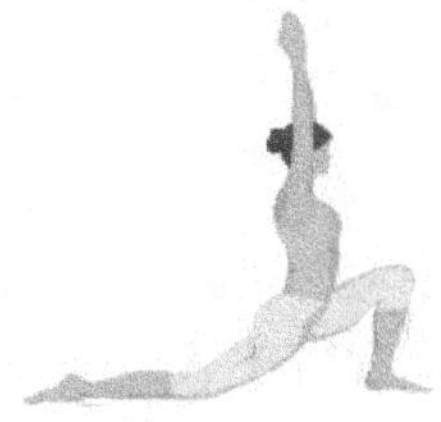

Previous Pose

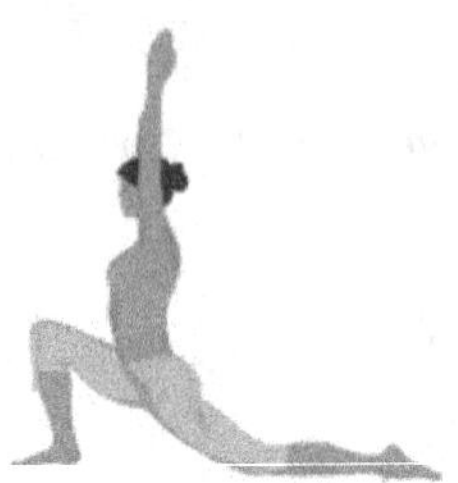

Anjaneyasana

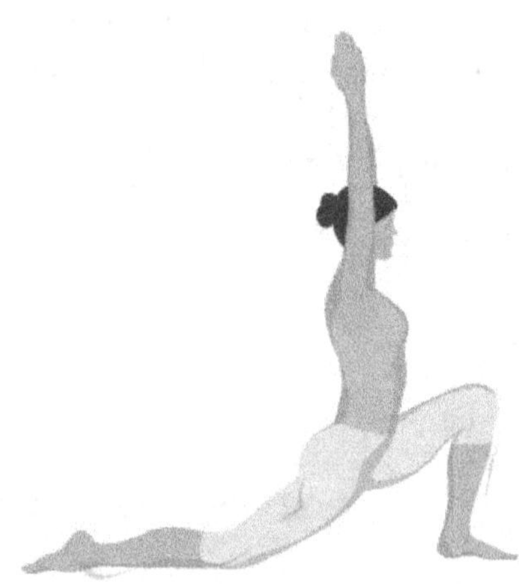

LOW LUNGE LEFT KNEE BENT AND FORWARD
#41

41. Low Lunge: Lizard: Left Knee Front and Bent
(Anjaneyasana)

1. Start in the downward dog pose.
2. Exhaling, step your left foot forward between your hands, with the sole flat on the floor.
3. The left knee is above the left ankle/heel.
4. Now lower your right knee towards the floor, so that the right knee and the right lower leg is now on the floor.
5. The right foot is sole upwards on the floor.
6. Slide backwards with the right leg if needed to get into a comfortable stretch – the left knee stays at 90 degrees bent position.
7. Now slowly raise both arms upwards so that they are perpendicular to the floor.
8. The biceps are touching both ears and the finger tips are pointing upwards.
9. Face forward- infinity. Hold this pose. Breathe normal.
10. Slowly bring your hands down and put your palms on the floor besides the left knee.
11. Pushing down on the palms, stretch your left leg backwards and slowly raising your torso, come into the downward facing dog pose.
12. Gradually lengthen your body and bring the chest and hips to the floor. You are now lying down with your arms by your side, palms down and your legs in a straight line with the spine and head. This is the reverse 'corpse' pose. From this position go to the sphynx pose.

Breathing: Normal during hold.

Gaze: Front infinity

Next Pose: Sphynx

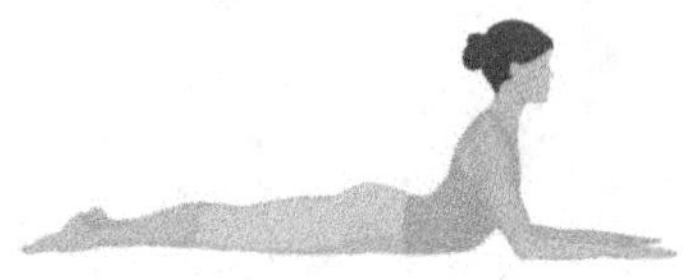

Previous Pose

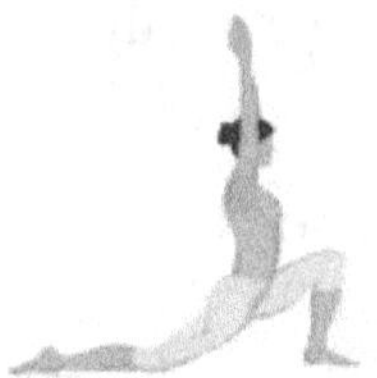

Salamba Bhujangasana

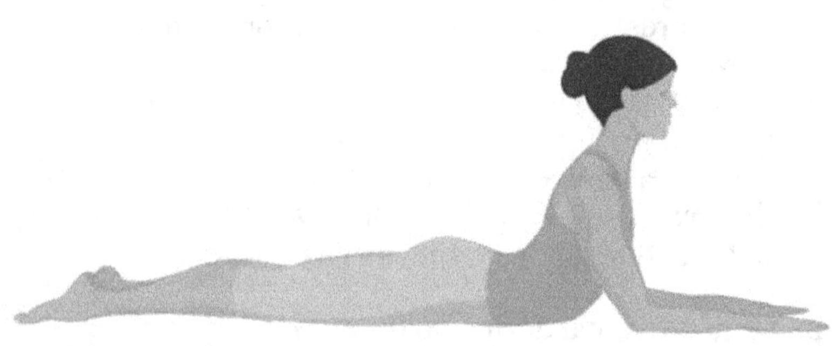

SPHYNX
#42

42. **Sphynx** *(Salamba Bhujangasana)*

1. From the face down position, slightly raising your upper torso, bring your elbows under your shoulders and your forearms on the floor parallel to each other. The hands are flat on the floor.
2. Inhale and lift your upper torso and head away from the floor into a mild backbend. Gaze straight forward to infinity.
3. Hold this pose. You can also put your head down straight or on either side for a resting position.

Breathing:

1. Inhalation during raising torso.
2. Normal breathing during hold

Gaze: Front/infinity

Transition pose: None

Next pose: Dolphin plank

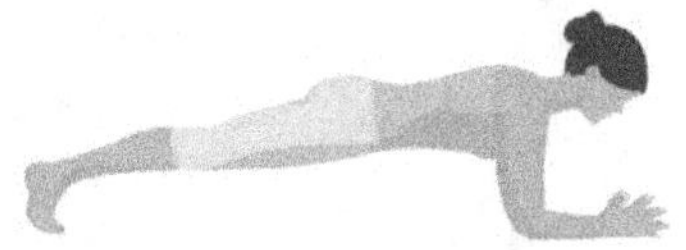

Previous Pose

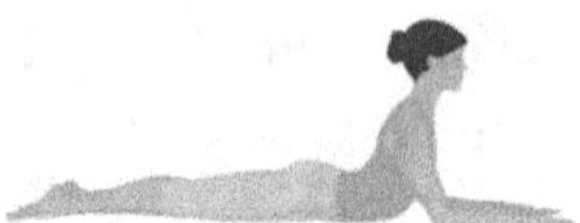

Makara Adho Mukha Svanasana

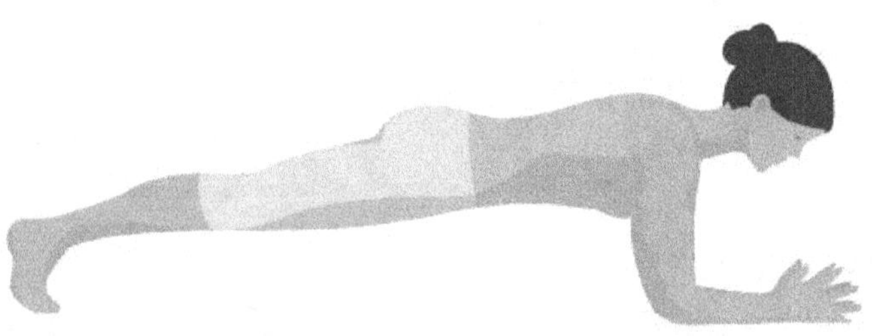

DOLPHIN PLANK
#43

43. **Dolphin Plank** *(Makara Adho Mukha Svanasana)*

1.   From the sphynx pose, lift your entire torso, with your feet on their toes.
2.   The forearms remain on the floor and the upper arms remain at right angles to the forearms
3.   The weight of the body is now resting on your forearms and toes.
4.   Your body should be flat and parallel to the floor. Your gaze should be at the floor.
5.   Hold pose. Breathe normally.
6.   Slowly lower yourself to the sphinx pose.

Breathing: Normal

Gaze: hands

Transition pose: Sphinx pose

Next pose: Cobra

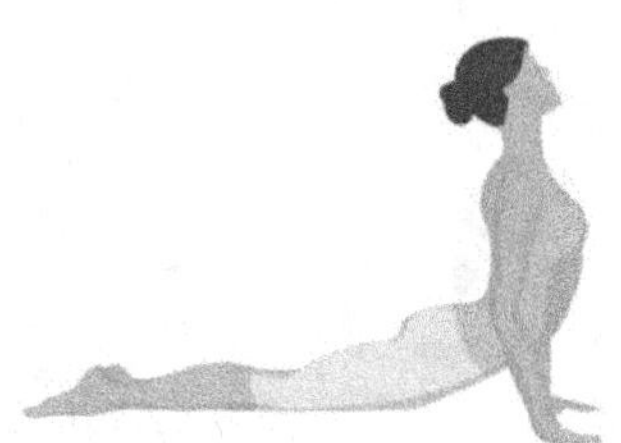

Previous Pose

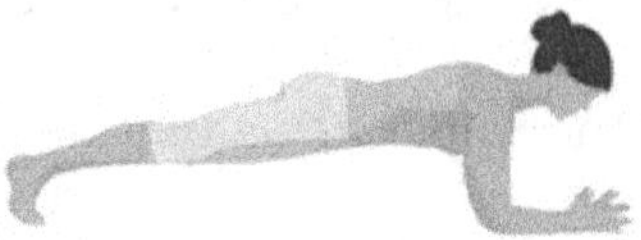

Bhujangasana

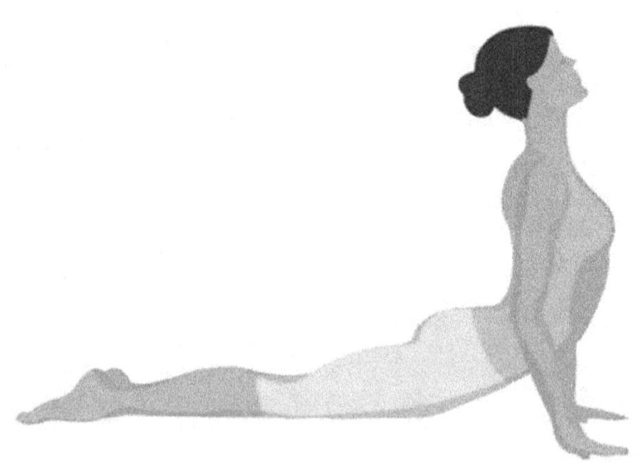

COBRA POSE
#44

44.Cobra *(Bhujangasana)*

1. Start from the sphinx pose.
2. Exhaling, press the tops of the feet and thighs and the pubis firmly into the floor.
3. Inhaling, gradually lift the chest and elbows off the floor. The groin should be touching the floor.
4. Raise your upper body to a comfortable height. The head and neck should be perpendicular to the floor.
5. Pull the shoulder blades backwards and towards each other while opening the chest in the front.
6. Gaze straight forward. Hold this pose.
7. Gradually lower yourself to the sphinx pose.

Breathing:

1. Rise up with inhalation
2. Normal breathing during hold

Gaze: Front/infinity

Transition pose: Sphinx pose

Next pose: Upward facing dog

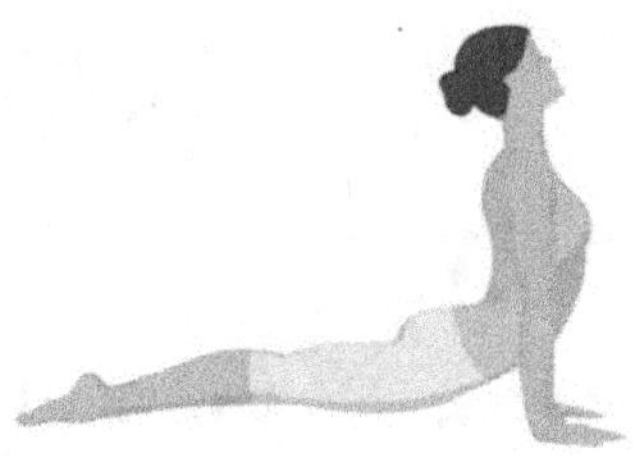

Previous Pose

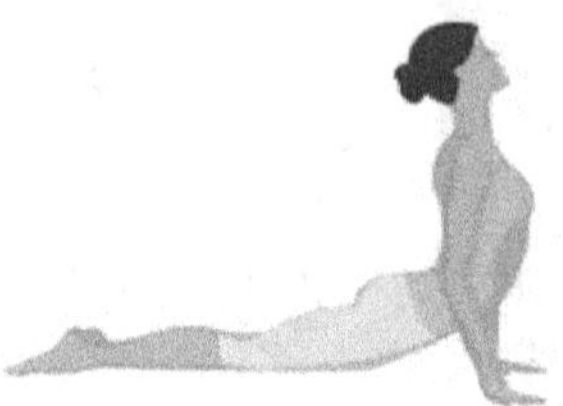

Urdhva Mukha Svanasana

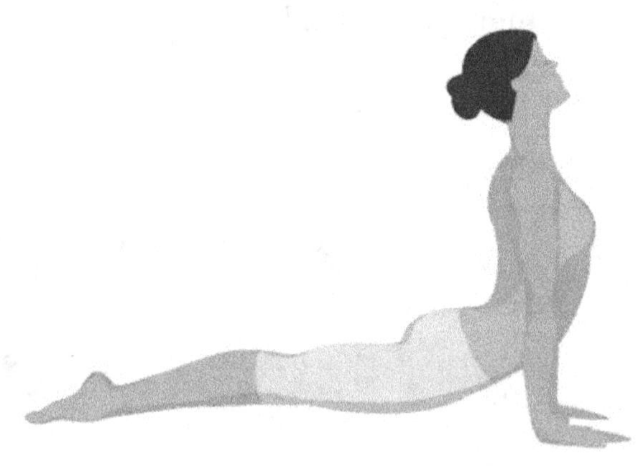

UPWARD FACING DOG
#45

45. **Upward Facing Dog** *(Urdhva Mukha Svanasana)*

1. From the sphinx pose, pressing against your feet (upper part of the feet should be firmly against the floor) slowly raise your upper body.
2. The arms gradually become perpendicular to the floor and the wrists and palms bear most of the weight of the upper torso. The palms are flat on the floor, with the finger tips facing forward.
3. Also raise the lower torso (including legs) off the floor so that the lower body weight is now mostly on the feet which have the tops touching the floor. Groin is off the floor.
4. Gaze forward. Hold position.
5. Move directly to the plank pose, unless you need rest. For rest - gradually lower yourself to the sphinx pose

Breathing: Raise the upper body during inhalation

Gaze: straight or up infinity

Transition pose: None

Next pose: Downward Facing Plank

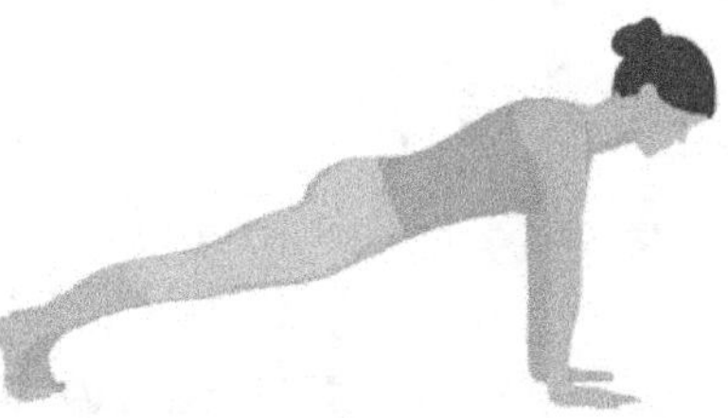

Previous Pose

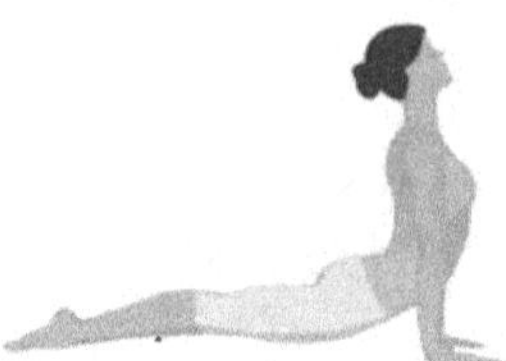

Phalakasana

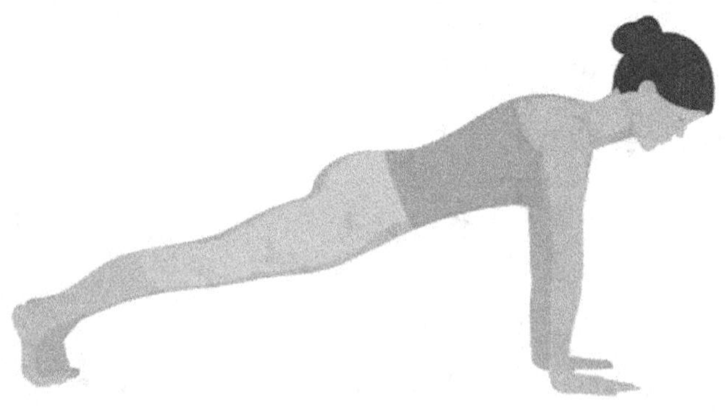

DOWNWARD PLANK
#46

46. Downward Facing Plank *(Phalakasana)*

1. From the upward facing dog, pull up and straighten your torso – so that the body is on the toes and the palms of the hands.
2. The arms are straight and shoulder apart.
3. The fingers of the hands are facing forward.
4. The entire torso should be straight and aligned.
5. Breathe normally during hold.

Breathing: Normal during hold

Gaze: Downwards at the hands

Transition pose: Sphynx

Next Pose: Locust

Previous Pose

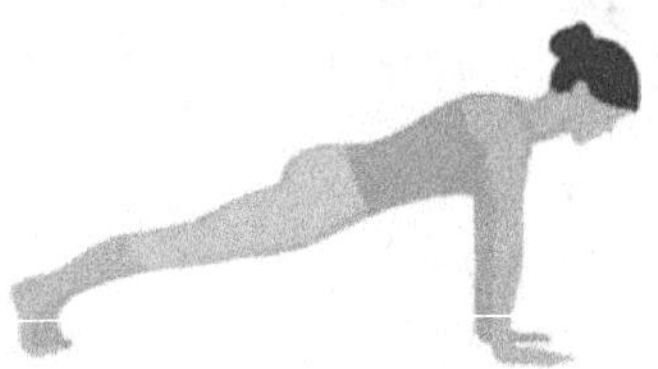

Salabhasana

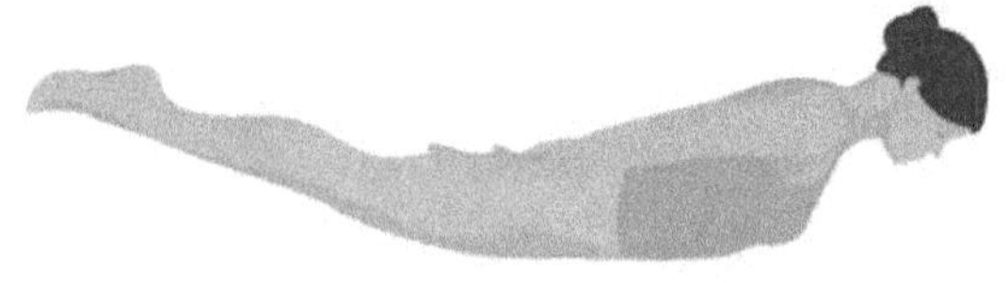

LOCUST POSE
#47

47. **Locust** *(Salabhasana)*

1. From the sphinx position, raise your head and upper torso to bring your arms by your side going backwards, and the palms resting besides your body on the floor.
2. Continue lifting your head and upper torso away from the floor. The upper body is now resting on your lower ribs and the belly.
3. Raise the legs away from the floor so the lower torso is resting on the lower pelvis and the feet, which are pointing back with the upper part of the feet against the floor. (soles facing up)
4. Gaze forward and hold pose
5. Gradually lower yourself back to the locust start pose.

Breathing: go into pose with inhalation

Gaze: floor/front

Transition pose: Sphynx

Next pose: Bow Pose

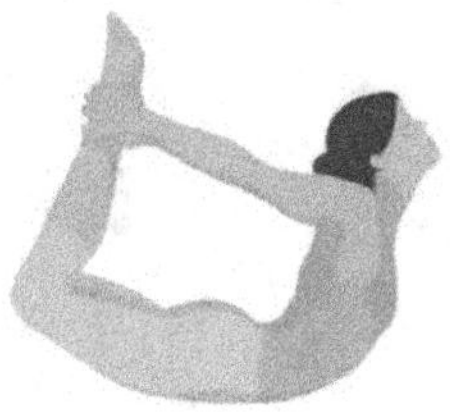

Previous Pose

Dhanurasana

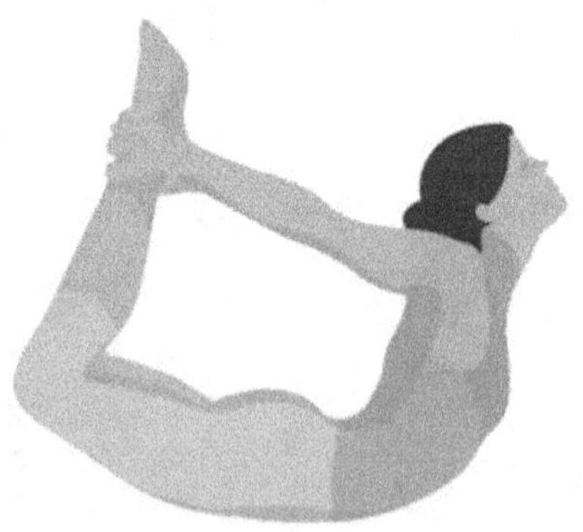

BOW POSE
#48

48. Bow *(Dhanurasana)*

1. From the locust start pose, slowly turn your palms facing upwards. The arms are still by your side and your body is resting on your torso. The feet are soles up with the toes pointing backwards.
2. Exhaling, bend your knees and bring your heels to the buttocks.
3. Inhaling, grab each ankle with your hands, with the knees being in line with your hips and not wider. Exhale. (It is ok if you cannot grab the legs in the beginning).
4. Inhaling, lift your thighs off the floor and at the same time lift your upper torso off the floor. Tighten the grip on the ankles.
5. You are now lying on the belly with the torso curved concave upwards.
6. Hold position Breathe normally. Gaze forward infinity
7. Exhaling, gradually lower yourself and rest in the sphinx pose.

Breathing: Go into pose with inhalation

Gaze: Straight/up infinity

Transition pose: None

Next pose: Reclining Buddha right

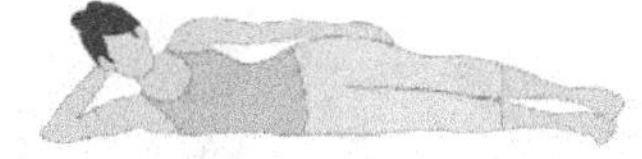

Previous Pose

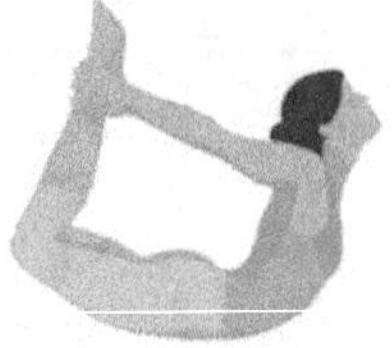

Mahaparinirvanasana

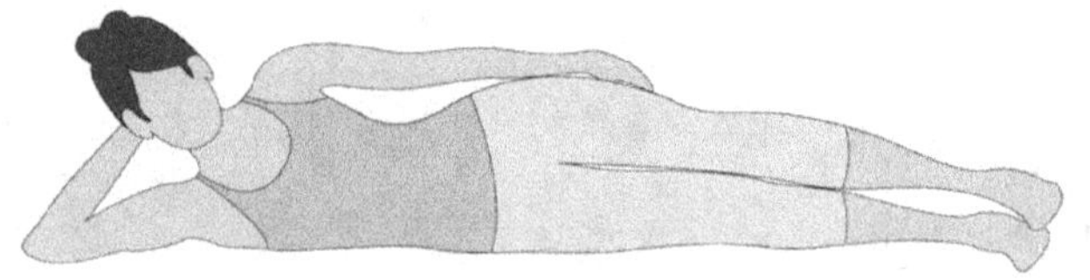

RECLINING BUDDHA RIGHT
#49

49. Reclining Buddha Right
(*Mahaparinirvanasana*)

1. From the sphinx pose, turn your body to the right, bringing your left arm alongside your upper side of your torso with the palm resting against the upper hip.
2. The left leg is on top of the right leg. The feet are perpendicular to the legs with the toes pointing forward.
3. At the same time, raise your head and neck and support them with the right arm. The upper arm rests on the floor while the lower arm is bent at right angles to the floor and supports the head in the palm of its hand.
4. The right palm is supporting the right jaw and the fingers are pointing towards the right ear.
5. Let the weight of your entire body fall on the torso touching the floor
6. Relax and hold this pose. Breathe normally.
7. Revert back to the sphinx pose.

Breathing: Normal during hold

Gaze: Front (right/facing side) infinity

Transition pose: None

Next pose: Side plank pose

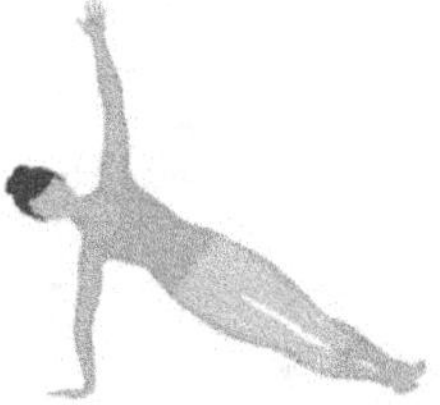

Previous Pose

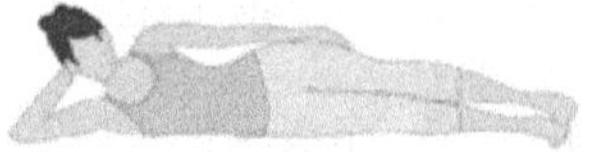

Vasisthansana

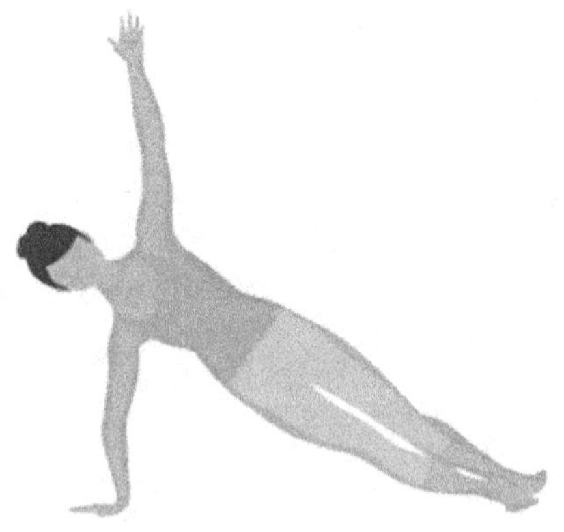

SIDE PLANK POSE RIGHT SIDE
#50

50.Side Plank: *(Vasisthasana)* **Right**

1. Turn your torso, so that you are resting on the right side of your body. Bring your left hand onto your right hip. At the same time, lift your upper body with your right hand, with the palm flat on the floor. Your rest of the lower body should be supported by the outer right foot.
2. Raise your left hand towards the ceiling.
3. The body should be off the floor except for the right palm and the right outer foot.
4. The torso should be in a straight stretched line from the toes to the crown.
5. The left leg should be resting on the right leg.
6. Hold pose. Gaze straight forward. Breathe normally.
7. Exhaling, come back to the sphinx pose.

Breathing:

1. Inhalation during raising of torso and arm.
2. Normal breathing during hold.

Gaze: Front (right/facing side) infinity

Transition pose: None

Next pose: Reclining Buddha left side

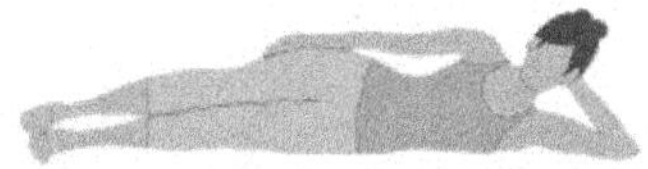

Previous Pose

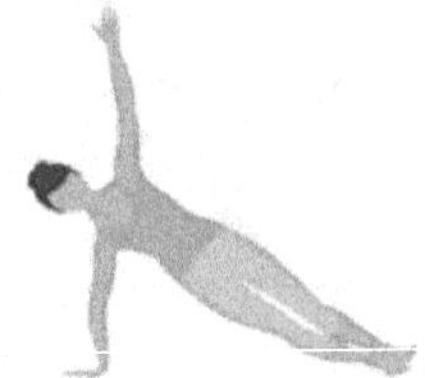

Mahaparinirvanasana

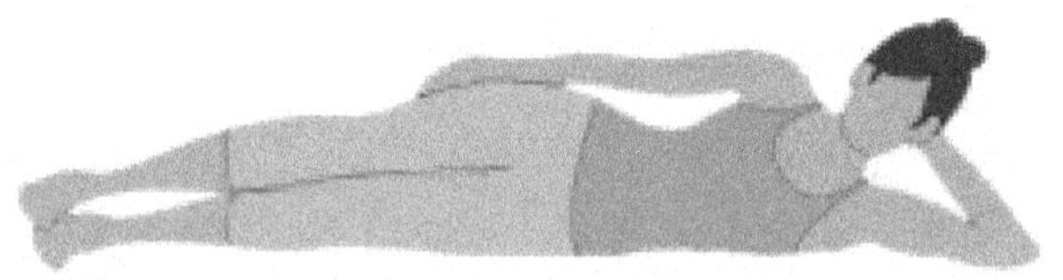

RECLINING BUDDHA LEFT SIDE
#51

51. Reclining Buddha: Left Side
(mahaparinirvanasana)

1. From the sphinx pose, turn your body to the left, bringing your right arm alongside your upper side of your torso with the palm resting against the upper hip.
2. The right leg is on top of the left leg. The feet are perpendicular to the legs with the toes pointing forward.
3. At the same time, raise your head and neck and support them with the left arm. The upper arm rests on the floor while the lower arm is bent at right angles to the floor and supports the head in the palm of its hand.
4. The left palm is supporting the left jaw and the fingers are pointing towards the left ear.
5. Let the weight of your entire body fall on the torso touching the floor
6. Relax and hold this pose. Breathe normally.
7. Revert back to the sphinx pose.

Breathing: Normal breathing during pose hold.

Gaze: Front (left side) infinity

Transition pose: None

Next pose: Side plank left

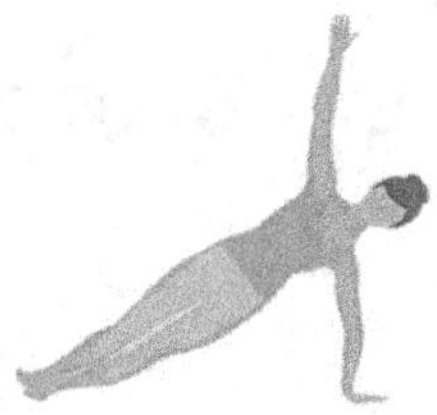

Previous Pose

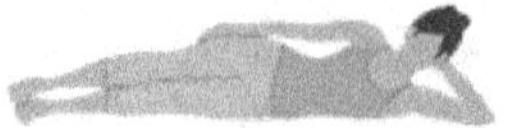

Vasisthansana

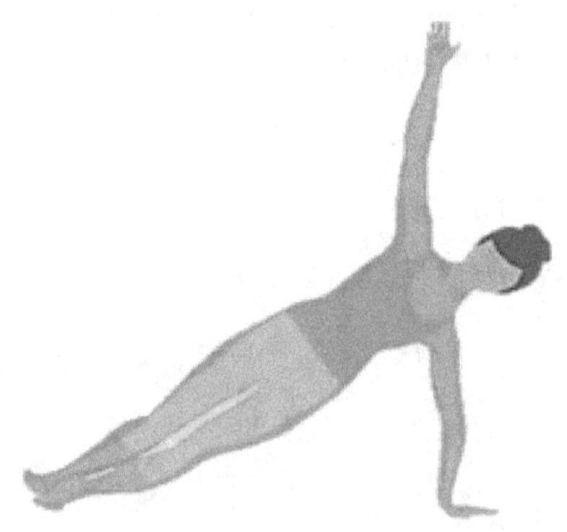

SIDE PLANK LEFT SIDE
#52

52. Side Plank: Left Side *(Vasisthasana)*

1. Turn your torso, so that you are resting on the left side of your body. Bring your right hand onto your left hip. At the same time, lift your upper body with your left hand, with the palm flat on the floor. Your rest of the lower body should be supported by the outer left foot.
2. Raise your right hand towards the ceiling.
3. The body should be off the floor except for the left palm and the left outer foot.
4. The torso should be in a straight stretched line from the toes to the crown.
5. The right leg should be resting on the left leg.
6. Hold this pose. Gaze straight forward. Breathe normally.
7. Exhaling, come back to the sphinx pose.
8. Now turn your body rightwards, and lay flat on your back, face up.

Breathing:

1. Inhalation during raising torso and arm.
2. Normal during hold.

Gaze: Forward (left side) infinity

Transition pose: None

Next pose: Corpse pose

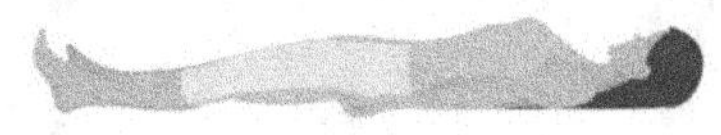

Previous Pose

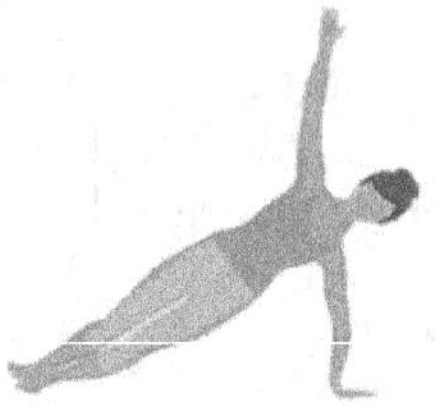

Savasana

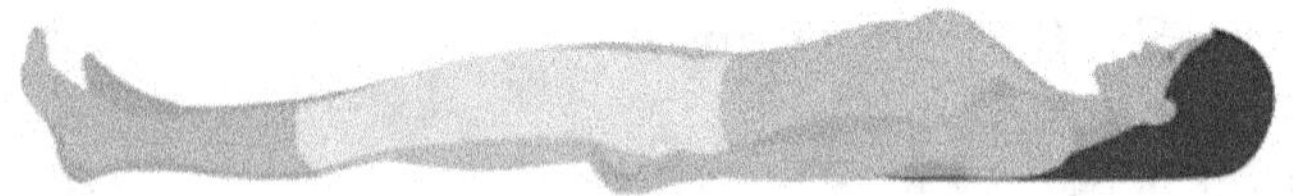

CORPSE POSE
#53

53. Corpse Pose *(savasana)*

1. After turning face up, ensure that your body is stretched, and your arms are by your side. Your entire body is resting against the ground.
2. The palms are facing up.
3. The legs which are on the floor, as is the torso and the head, normally rotate out with the toes facing up and away from each other.
4. Make sure you are in a 'neutral' position with no tension.
5. Breathe nice and easy through the nostrils.
6. Gaze is upwards infinity.

Breathing: Normal

Gaze: upwards/infinity

Transition pose: None

Next pose: Half boat to full boat pose

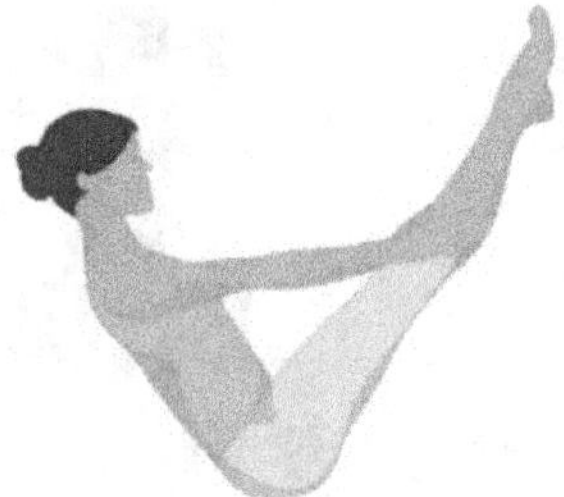

Previous Pose

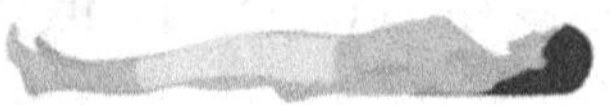

Navasana

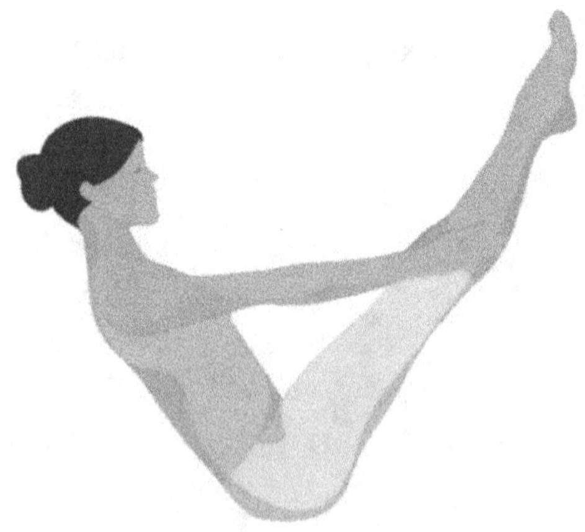

BOAT POSE
#54

54. Boat Pose *(Navasana)*

1. From the corpse pose (face up), sit up, pushing with the hands and arms. The palms are flat on the floor. Now bend your knees 90 degrees and perpendicular to the floor. Bring your feet, with the soles against the floor and with the palms flat on the ground, as close to the buttocks as possible.
2. Now, slowly lean back slightly, keeping your spine straight.
3. Lift your feet off the ground and bring your shins parallel to the floor.
4. Sitting on the back bone, lift your hands off the floor and bring the arms parallel to the floor, on either side of the legs, with the palms facing towards each other.
5. The spine should remain straight.
6. This is half boat. Hold this pose.
7. Now straighten your legs so the that feet are now pointing up and the legs are at an angle of 45 degree from the ground. The body now assumes a 'V' shape.
8. This is the full boat pose. Hold this pose.
9. Gradually bring your arms and legs down and assume the corpse pose.

Breathing: Normal breathing during the hold.

Gaze: Legs/feet

Transition pose: Corpse pose

Next pose: Happy baby pose

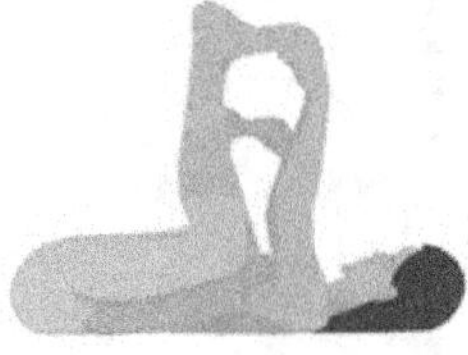

Previous Pose

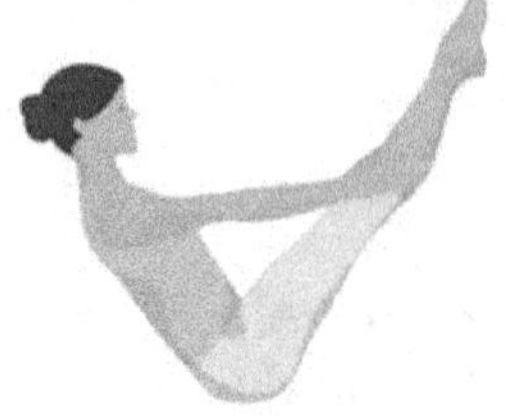

Ananda Balasana

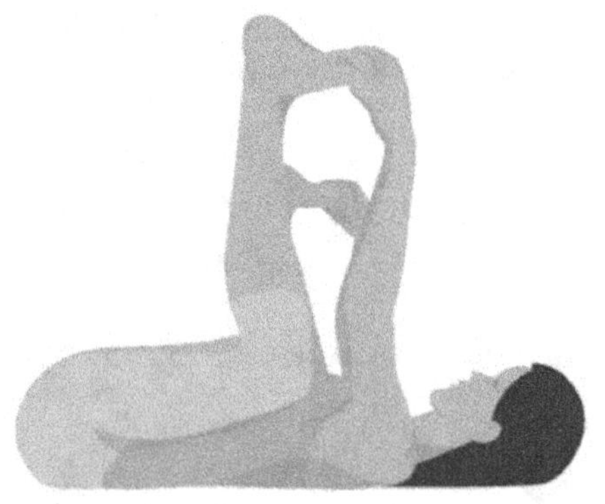

HAPPY BABY POSE

#55

55. **Happy Baby Pose** *(Ananda Balasana)*

1. Start in the *savasana* pose.
2. Exhaling, bend your knees, bringing them close to your belly.
3. Inhaling, grasp each ankle with the corresponding hand.
4. Now raise the ankles upwards, spreading out the knees and bringing them closer to the armpits. The lower legs should now be perpendicular to the floor. The ankles should be directly above your knees.
5. Slide your hands to the feet and flex them slightly. The arms are straight upwards.
6. The head should continue resting on the floor.
7. Hold pose. Breathe normally.
8. Return gently to the corpse pose.

Breathing: Normal during hold

Gaze: Toes

Transition pose: Corpse pose

Next pose: Wind relief pose

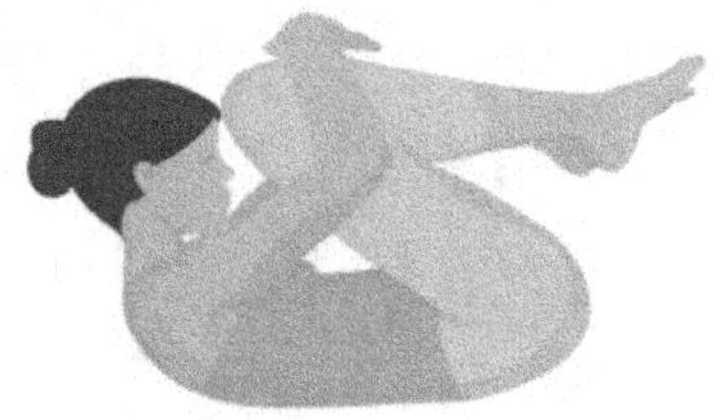

Previous Pose

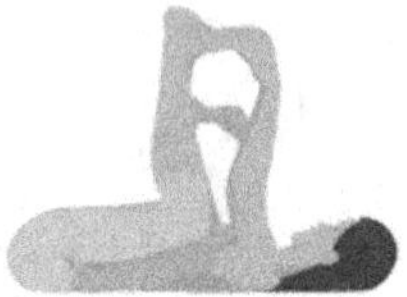

Pavanamuktasana

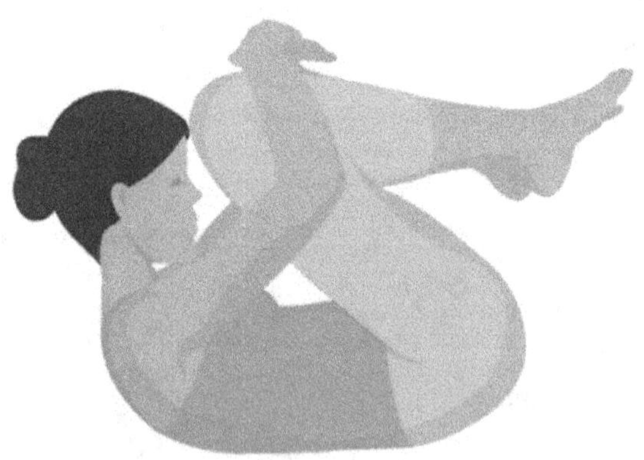

WIND RELIEF POSE
#56

56. Wind Relief Pose *(Pavanamuktasana)*

1. Start in the corpse pose.
2. Exhaling, bring both of your knees towards your chin, against the chest. Clasp your hands around them. If you cannot clasp your hands around the legs, hold on to the upper legs but make sure the legs are firmly against each other.
3. Holding firm to the legs in this pose, slowly roll your body from head to lower back. Do this ten times.
4. It is normal to pass gas during this process – hence the name.
5. Letting go the hands, slowly bring the legs and feet down.
6. Return to the corpse pose.

Breathing:

1. Exhalation during bending the knees towards the chest.
2. Normal breathing through hold. Inhalation on returning to corpse pose.

Gaze: Knees

Transition pose: Corpse Pose

Next pose: Bridge pose

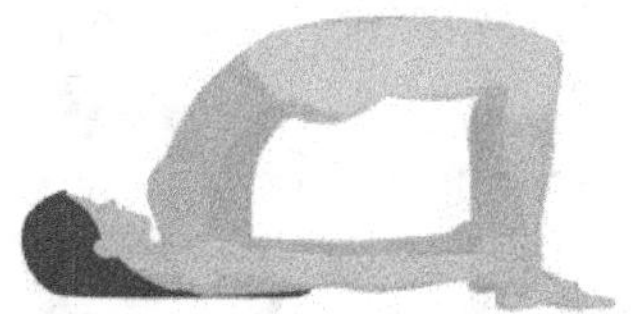

Previous Pose

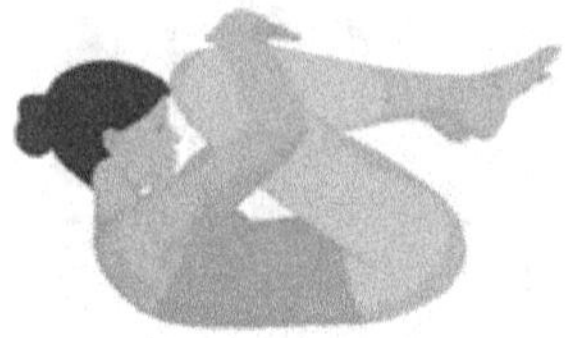

Setubandha

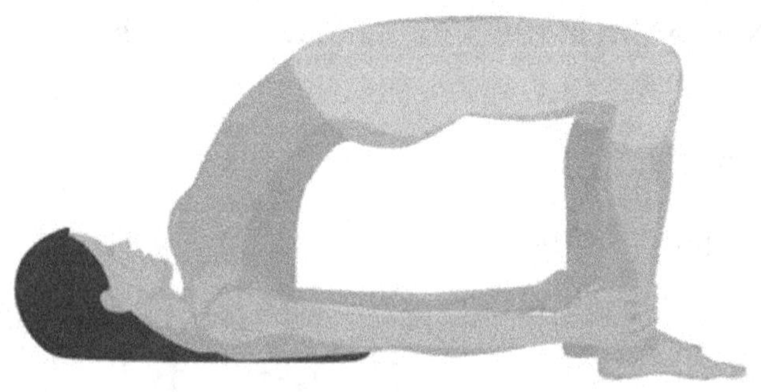

BRIDGE POSE
#57

57. **Bridge Pose** *(Setubandha)*

1. From the corpse pose, bend your knees and bring them as close to the buttocks as possible.
2. Press on your palms and feet downwards and inhaling lift your buttocks in the air towards the pubic bone.
3. The lower legs should be perpendicular to the floor now and the thighs and feet aligned in a straight line.
4. The knees should be above the ankles.
5. Lift your shoulder blades pushing your sternum upwards.
6. Bring your hands under your torso and clasp them together.
7. The head and feet stay flat on the floor.
8. Gaze is upwards infinity. Hold pose. Breathe normally.
9. Return to the corpse pose

Breathing:

1. Inhalation during trunk lift.
2. Normal breathing during hold.
3. Exhalation on return to corpse pose.

Gaze: Ceiling/upwards infinity

Transition pose: Corpse Pose

Next pose: Back Plank

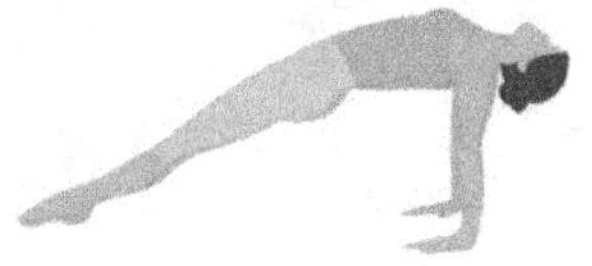

Previous Pose

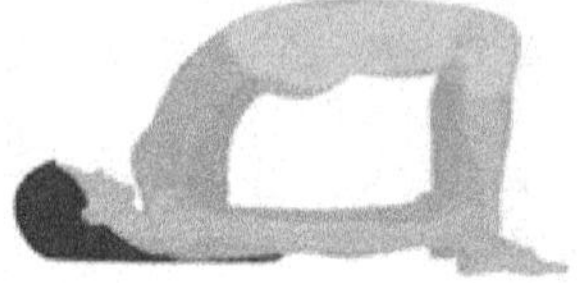

Purvottanasana

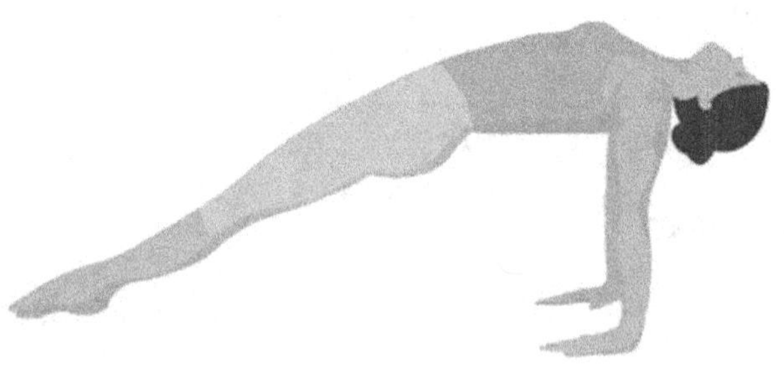

BACK PLANK
#58

58. Upward (Back Plank) *(Purvottanasana)*

1. Sit up to the *dandasana* pose – legs straight in front of you and torso erect at right angles to the thighs/floor.
2. Move your hands palms down against the floor – behind your hips with the fingers pointing forwards.
3. Exhaling, lift your torso while pushing down on your hands and feet against the floor.
4. Stretch your torso and slowly drop your head backwards. The palms and feet stay flat on the floor.
5. Hold this pose. Breathe normally.
6. Slowly lower yourself to the corpse pose.

Breathing:

1. Inhalation during lifting of torso.
2. Normal during hold.

Gaze: Upwards infinity

Transition pose: Corpse pose

Next pose: Both Knee Bend Pose: Right Side

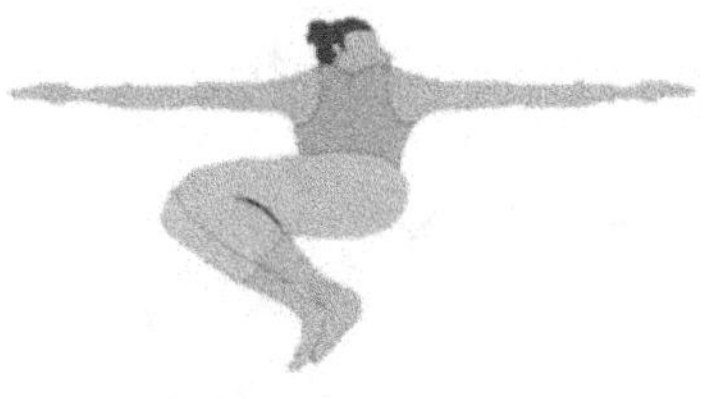

Previous Pose

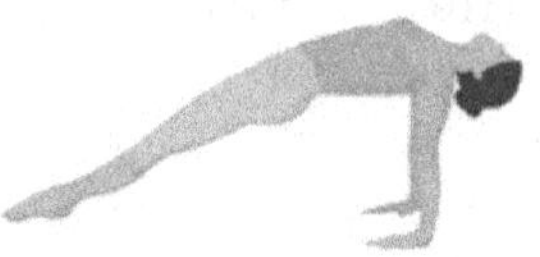

Jathara Parivartanasana

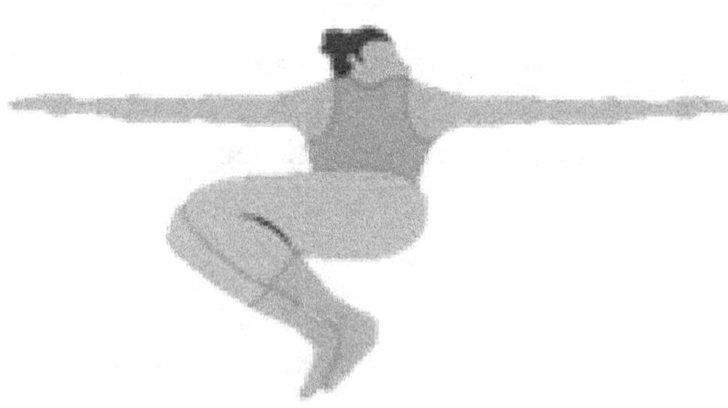

SUPINE SPINAL TWIST RIGHT SIDE
#59

59. Supine Spinal Twist – Revolved Abdominal Pose: Right Side *(Jathara Parivartanasana)*

1. From the corpse pose, bend your knees and keep the soles flat on the floor.
2. Extend arms to a T position. (If there is not enough space to extend the arms, bring the right arm to the right thigh, holding it if possible; the left arm can go across your chest)
3. Lower legs down to the right, with the right knee touching the ground. Turn your head to the left.
4. Bring knees to center. Extend knees to return to the corpse pose.

Breathing:

1.   Exhalation during twist
2.   Normal breathing during hold
3.   Inhalation during return to corpse pose

Gaze: Left thumb

Transition pose: Corpse pose

Next pose: Supine spinal twist – revolved abdominal pose

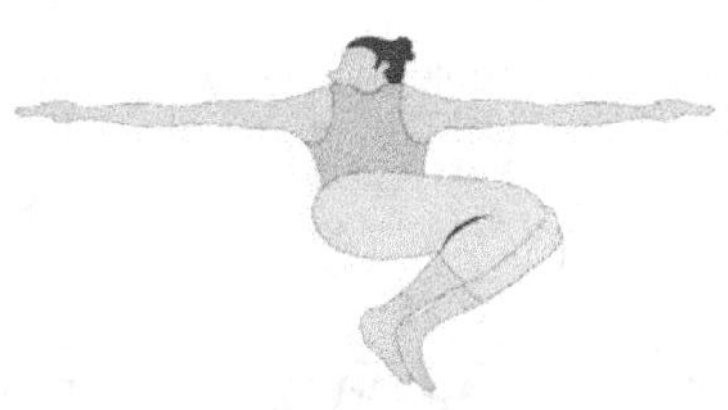

Previous Pose

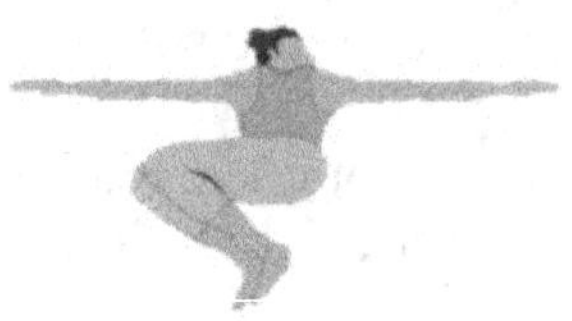

Jathara Parivartanasana

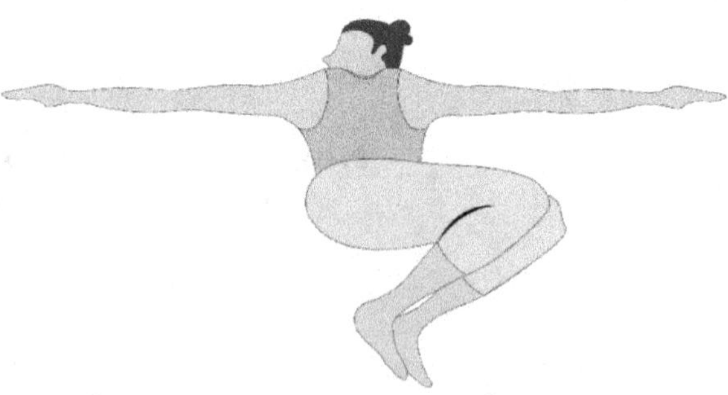

SUPINE SPINAL TWIST LEFT SIDE
#60

60. Supine Spinal Twist – Revolved Abdominal Pose: Left Side *(Jathara Parivartanasana)*

1. From the corpse pose, bend your knees and keep the soles flat on the floor.
2. Extend arms to a T position. (If there is not enough space to extend the arms, bring the right arm to the right thigh, holding it if possible; the left arm can go across your chest)
3. Lower legs down to the left, with the left knee touching the ground. Turn your head to the right.
4. Bring knees to center. Extend knees to return to the corpse pose.

Breathing:

    1. Exhalation during twist
    2. Normal breathing during hold
    3. Inhalation during return to corpse pose

Gaze: Right thumb

Final pose: Corpse pose

Next pose: Supine Stretch in Corpse pose

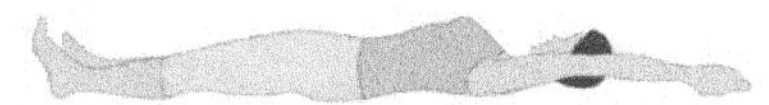

Previous Pose

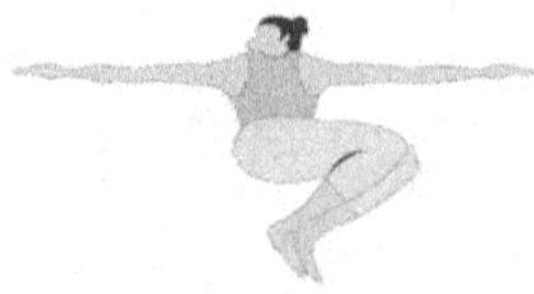

Supta uttanasana

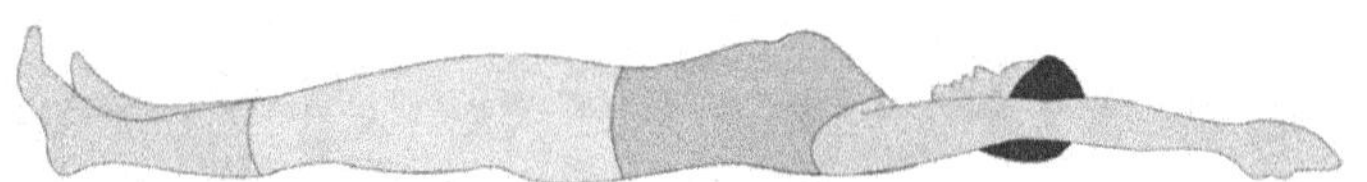

SUPINE STRETCH
Final Pose

Final: *Savasana* to **Supine Stretch** *(Supta uttanasana)*

1. In the corpse pose, inhaling, stretch your arms over your head, but still touching the floor. They should remain parallel to each other. Exhale.
2. Inhaling again, stretch the entire body as if being pulled by the hands in one direction and pulled by the feet in the other direction. Stay aligned and in contact with the floor.
3. Hold position. Breather normally during the hold phase. Gaze is upwards to the ceiling
4. Exhaling, gradually relax and return to the corpse pose.

Breathing:

1. Inhalation during stretch
2. Normal breathing during hold
3. Exhalation on returning back to corpse pose

Gaze: Ceiling/upwards infinity

Final Relaxing Pose: Corpse pose

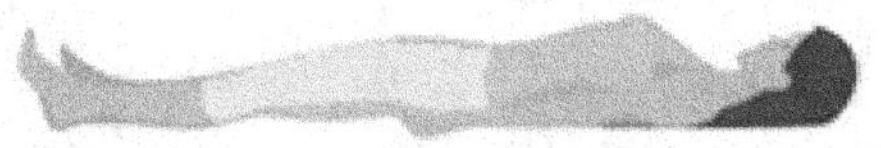

b. Total body relaxation

Now go through a process of whole body relaxation while in the corpse (*savasana*) pose. This will ready your body for the breathing exercises. Consciously focus, with the eyes closed, on the left toe and will it to be relaxed. Now move up to the whole left foot, then the ankle, to the left lower leg, the left knee and the left upper leg – consciously encouraging the muscles to relax completely. They should be completely tension free. Move up to the left hip, left side of the pelvis, left abdomen, left side of the chest, left shoulder, left upper arm, left elbow, left forearm and left hand and fingers. Relax each section as you move on. Now come back up to the left side of the neck, left side of the face and left side of the head and start heading down the right side of the head to the right face and reversing the entire sequence from the right arm, right side of the torso, right leg and finally to the right toes. The whole body should be now completely relaxed and feel like a log on the ground. This is the true *savasana* - or corpse pose. Breathe quietly through your nostrils, feeling the air on the nostril tips, and try to keep your mind thought free. Stay in this pose for a few minutes before opening your eyes and starting the breathing exercises.

REMEMBER....

Do the best you can. This is not a competitive sport. There is nothing to prove to yourself or others. Do the poses to the extent they are comfortable. Do not invite pain. West says, 'no pain no gain'. Yoga says: 'pain means no gain'. Yoga exercises done diligently will make you realize that you actually get better as you get older - and your endurance increases – unlike many other workouts. So, do what you can - enjoy the stillness and peace accruing from this yoga routine. You will also become a better person - for yourself and for the universe.

As mentioned before, physical activity or physical exercise is measured in METs. One MET is approximately equal to a person's resting energy expenditure (e.g. sitting quietly in a chair) Physical activity is categorized into three categories: light-intensity activities are defined as 1.1 MET to 2.9 METs; moderate-intensity activities are defined as 3.0 to 5.9 METs and vigorous-intensity activities are defined as 6.0 METs or more. Larson-Meyer reviewed 17 studies and concluded that METs for individual asanas averaged 2.2 ± 0.7 – low intensity, whereas that of pranayamas was 1.3 ± 0.3 – also low intensity. Yoga practice (not including sun salutations) is therefore generally considered as a low intensity exercise.

"... a timeless state where there is no death or birth or growth, where there is no pain or sorrow, where there is no day or night, nor any distance........such a state can be achieved by meditating upon the self within, and realizing that I am everywhere and in everything."

Swami Vishnu-Devananda

c. **Breathing Exercises** *(Pranayama)*

"God is the breath inside the breath"

Kabir

Disturbed physical and emotional health are not conducive to proper breathing. You tend to breathe shallower and faster. Yoga says that breath contains more than air - you breathe 'prana' (good energy) on inhalation and you discard 'apana' (bad energy) on exhalation.

'Prana' is not oxygen or any other physical constituents of the air - prana is universal energy. An energy that is present in everything in this cosmos. Pranayama or breathing exercises that help you regulate and recharge our 'pranic' batteries by connecting to this inexhaustible energy source. The fresh infusion of vital cosmic energy will lead to a noticeable physical and mental rejuvenation. Similarly, exhalation is associated with elimination of 'apana' - the unhealthy and often toxic energy generated and accumulating in your body.

Breathing is vital to life. It has been said that you are given a limited number of breaths in our life - use them fast and you leave this body earlier - use them slowly and you keep our body longer. An example is often cited from the animal kingdom - rabbits who breathe fast have short lives while some breeds of tortoises may breathe only once a minute and can live hundreds of years. The first breath jump starts your life and the last breath terminates it.

Most people in the modern world breathe improperly and inefficiently. We subconsciously train ourselves to chest breathing- a breathing pattern conducive to prolonged sitting - in car, sofa or at worked. This breathing is restricted, usually limited to the middle chest. There is hardly any abdominal movement during such breathing. It is often associated with stress and anxiety and results in a faster shallower breathing and a fast heart rate. However, if you watch babies when they are sleep - they perform abdominal breathing. This is the natural form of breathing that is good for our health. Many of us also perform abdominal breathing during sleep. The purpose of yoga is to teach the technique of a proper breathing, which with repetition lowers your breathing rate, improves your breathing capacity and exercises all the numerous muscles, ligaments and bones involved with respiration (besides the diaphragm).

The yogic view of breathing goes beyond that taught by schools of anatomy and physiology. The yogis believe that when we breathe in, we inhale (besides oxygen containing air) unseen and unfelt 'prana'. 'Prana' is cosmic energy - an unseen force that is pervasive in life. Inhaling 'prana' with the first breath kick starts life outside the womb. When 'prana' leaves the body, we die. During our life 'prana' sustains life. The level of 'prana' and the quality of 'prana' we have determines our life – a life of vigor or sluggishness, a life of either misery or happiness and so on. The yogis believe that this pranic energy can be increased and its quality improved, by controlling the quantity and quality of breaths we take - controlled yogic breathing. This also helps remove 'apana' - the unhealthy and often toxic energy created and ending up being stored in our bodies.

Pranic energy is said to be stored in the solar plexus - an 'abdominal brain'. The concept of an abdominal brain may be underlying the phrases, 'sick to my stomach' or 'butterflies in my stomach' - phrases not related to food or gastric function. Proper 'prana' circulates throughout the body through thousands of channels called 'nadis' (invisible passageways akin to the Chinese acupuncture meridians). The smooth and unrestricted flow of this vital energy is often interrupted by blocks called 'granthis' along the 'nadis'. Proper breathing via breathing exercises helps remove these obstacles and allows a smooth flow of cosmic energy all over our body. Yogis also believe that there is an unlimited amount of good energy stored in our 'kundilini', and this can flow upwards through a channel in your spine called the 'sushuma', towards your brain, if released. This energy is often also blocked at various levels – which can be opened up. The kundalini energy can rise and get stuck at seven energy centers – called 'chakras'

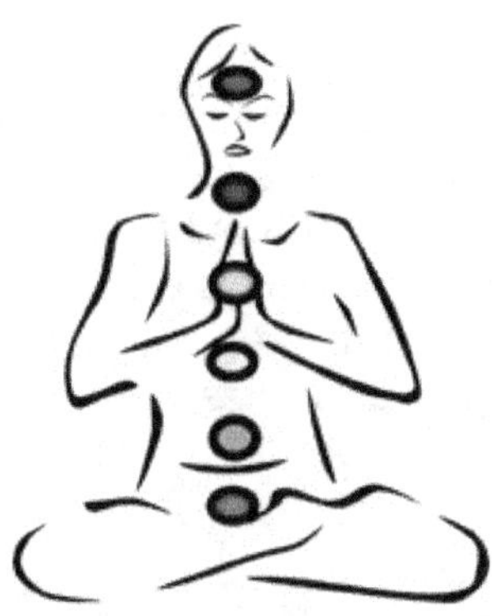

These are:

Root Center (*Mulathara Chakra*): This is located at the base of the spine. It is associated with basic survival instincts and actions.

Naval Center (*Swadhisthana Chakra*): This is located in the lower abdomen, approximately two inches below the naval and two inches inward. It is associated with sexuality.

Solar Plexus Center (*Manipura Chakra*): Located in the upper abdomen, just below the breast bone. It is an ego center, dealing with self-worth, self-confidence, self-esteem and power.

Heart Center (*Anahata Chakra*): Located in the center of the chest and associated with the heart, it deals with feelings and actions of love, compassion and inner joy.

Throat Center (*Visuddha Chakra*): As the name indicates, it is located in the throat area. It deals with communication - expression of feelings.

Brow Center (*Ajna Chakra*): It is located between the eyebrows and behind. It is associated with intuition, wisdom, imagination.

Crown Center (*Shasraha Chakra*): Located at the top of the head. It represents universal beauty, spiritual illumination and pure bliss. (not highlighted in the picture above)

The center to which this kundalini energy rises and gets stuck often characterizes you - for example, if this energy is stuck at the solar plexus level, you are egoistic in all aspects - demanding power and control. If your kundalini energy rises to your heart level – you will radiate love and compassion. Breathing exercises over a period of time can help release these blocks and allow the kundilini energy to rise, improving your character and ultimately granting us internal peace and bliss.

Remember,

"A reduction of 'prana' or an excess accumulation of 'apana' can cause a serious disruption to the flow of our physical, mental and spiritual energies. Pranayama exercises can help unblock these obstacles, allowing for the free flow on good energy and the expedited removal of bad energy - thereby helping restore a healthy cosmic balance in our bodies and soul."

Before you learn breath control and exercises, spend some time becoming aware of your breathing. Sense your breath entering in your body via your nostrils and sense it leaving your body via your nostrils. The entire inspiration should be smooth (not stuttered) and calm (not strenuous) - the breath should feel like a 'silky' air movement' softly caressing your nostrils. Similarly, after a short natural pause, the expiration should also be smooth and relaxed, impairing the same silky touch to your nostril tips. Breath awareness is essential to master - it is to be noticed and controlled during asanas and also during meditation. Sitting or lying down in a quiet atmosphere and monitoring your smooth silky breath for about 10 cycles is a daily exercise, that should become routine on waking up and before going to sleep. It will also be incorporated with yoga postures, practiced before and after breathing exercises and before, during and after meditation. No sounds should be produced during breathing and the whole experience should be calming and peaceful.

I recommend you learn the following breathing techniques and exercises:

1. Complete breath (technique)
2. Complete breath with holds. (exercise)
3. Complete breath with locks. (exercise)
4. Alternate nostril breathing. (exercise)

5. Core massaging breathing. (exercise)
6. Silk breath. (relaxation)

Total time: 10 minutes

Place and time for breathing exercises:

Place:

The ideal place to do the yogic breathing is:

1. Comfortable sitting or lying place - sitting on a soft yoga mat or lying in bed. If nothing is available, a folded sheet or towel should suffice.
2. Quiet environment without distractions from people, radio, tv or cell phones.
3. Not too bright or too dark. Early morning hours or early evening hours are good.
4. Soft slow beat music in the background - if available. Your headphones with soft music playing close to you may do the job.
5. Light fragrance in the air - fresh flowers or incense or other source of perfume.
6. You may keep a watch close by although I strongly recommend that you count your seconds mentally. This will further help you block out external distractions and internal thoughts.

Time:

You should not be on a full stomach. You should be calm and relaxed. These exercises can be otherwise done anytime – and literally anywhere.

Preferred postures for breathing exercises:

1. **Sitting - Easy pose** *(Sukhasana)*

   1. Breathing normally, lower your torso, place both hands on the floor, sit down on your buttocks and straighten out the legs in front of you.
   2. Sit up straight. (This is the *dandasana* pose)
   3. Cross your legs in front of you and fold them near your torso.

4. With the knees wide apart, tuck your feet beneath the opposite knee. Either shin can be on top – it is good to alternate on different days. The position should be easy and relaxed.
5. Place your palms on the knees, facing down or up, and without any tension. Adopt a mudra that you feel comfortable with. (breathing mudras described after these poses)
6. Hold this pose. Gaze is front infinity. Breathe normally. This is also a rest position.

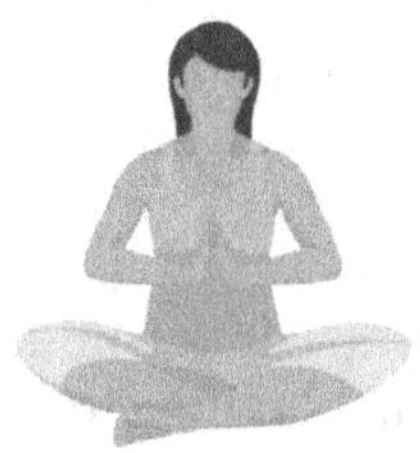

2. **Sitting - Half lotus pose** (*Ardha Padmasana*)

1. Sit on the floor with the torso straight up and the legs stretched perpendicular forwards, parallel to each other and on the floor.
2. Bend the right knee and pull up the right ankle to the top of your left hip.
3. Bend your left knee and push your left ankle below the left knee
4. Rest your hands on the knees and adopt a mudra you like.

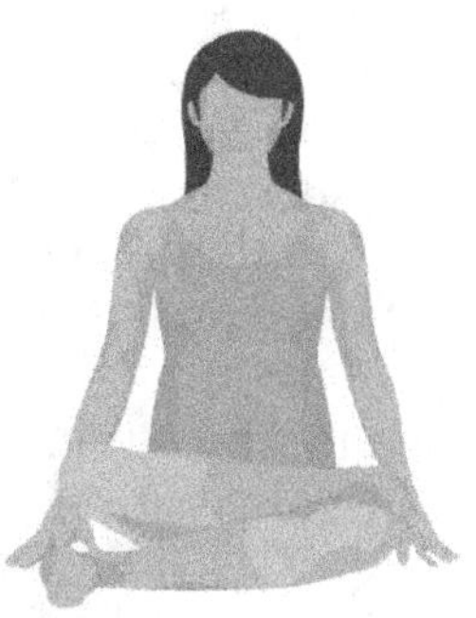

3. **Sitting - Lotus pose** *(Padmasana)*

1. Breathing normally, lower your torso, place both hands on the floor, sit down on your buttocks and straighten out the legs in front of you.
2. Sit up straight. (This is the *dandasana* pose)
3. Bending your right knee bring it towards your chest and lower it to the front crease of the left hip. The foot will be turned facing up – the sole of the foot faces upwards.
4. Do the same thing with the left knee and ankle. The left lower leg and ankle go over the right shin and rest on the right hip crease.
5. The knees should be close together and you should be sitting up straight.
6. Rest your hands on the knees. Adopt a mudra as desired.

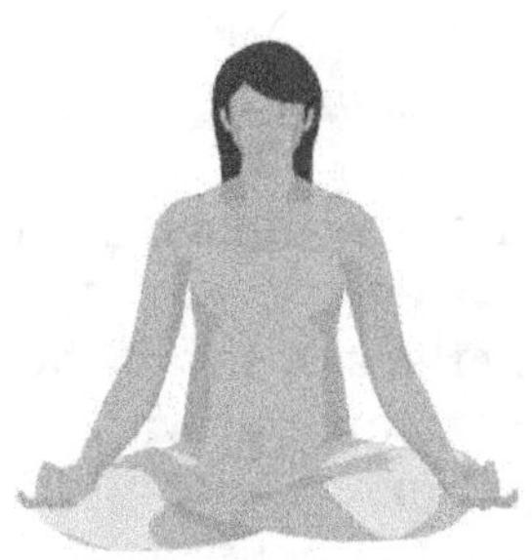

4. Sitting - Hero pose *(Virasana)*

1.   From the mountain *(tadasana)* pose, inhaling, bend forward, lower your body and place your knees on the floor. The legs go backwards perpendicular to the thighs but parallel to each other on the floor. Your torso and head are straight up, in line with the thighs.
2.   Place your hands on the thighs. Sit back in between the two legs. Your position should be snug with the outer thighs in contact with your inner calves.
4.   Chest should be straight up with the face looking forward. Gaze would be front infinity.
5.   Hold position. Breathe normally. This is also a rest position. If you are unable to sit on the floor, sit on a folded blanket placed in between your thighs/feet.
6.   Adopt a hand mudra according to your preference.

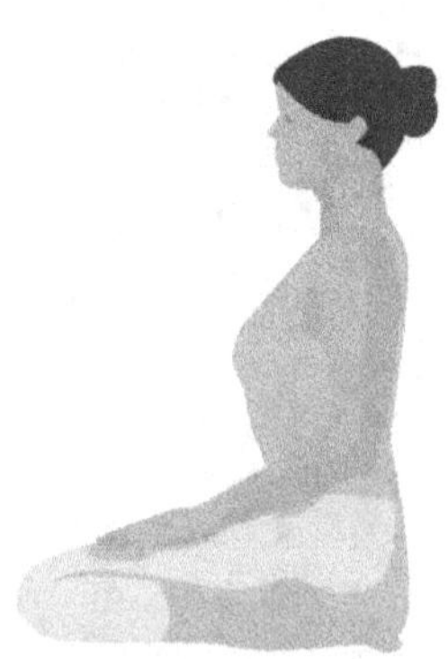

5. Corpse pose *(Savasana)*

1.   Lie down on the floor with face up. The entire body should be aligned and relaxed.
2.   Bring the arms by the sides with the palms facing up.
3.   The legs normally rotate out with the toes facing up and away from each other.
4.   Make sure you are in a 'neutral' position with no tension.
5.   Breathe nice and easy through the nostrils.

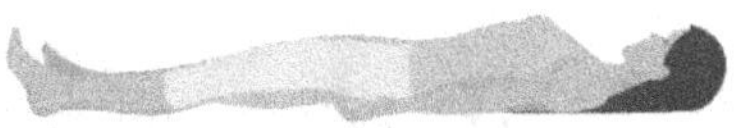

Mudra (hand gestures) for breathing:

Hand gestures are often applied during breathing exercises. The hands are thought to represent different areas of the body (Chinese acupuncture/acupressure) and proper alignment facilitates specific breathing patterns. The ancient yogis also postulate energy flowing from the chakras (energy centers) and hand gestures allow this energy to be retained inside the body by particular hand gestures (closing the fist or forming a circle with fingers prevents the energy from escaping)

The hand gestures commonly applied during the breathing exercises while sitting require the hands to rest on each knee. These mudras include:

1. **Chin Mudra:** The tips of the thumb and first finger (index finger) made to touch each other forming an oval space. The palms are facing upwards. The other three fingers are extended (kept straight). The hands should be relaxed. This mudra encourages and facilitates abdominal breathing by focusing on diaphragmatic movements.

2. **Chinmaya Mudra:** The tips of the thumb and index finger are touching each other and positioned the same way as in Chin mudra. The palm is facing up. The other three fingers are however curled inwards and folded on the palm. This mudra is conducive to the use of the intercostal muscles and chest breathing. The chest opens sideways.

3. **Adhi Mudra:** In this gesture, the hand is formed into a fist. The thumb is first folded on the palm with the tip towards the little finger. The rest of the fingers then curl over the thumb and cover

it, forming a firm yet relaxed fist. This mudra is associated with clavicular or upper chest breathing. The chest opens forwards with this mudra.

4. **Brahma Mudra:** With both fists folded as in Adhi mudra, bring them together in the middle of the lap with the knuckles touch flat against each other and the closed palms facing up. The thumb is facing forward and the little fingers touching the abdomen. This mudra is great for complete breath.

I suggest you use the Brahma mudra during your sitting breathing exercises. If these mudras attract unwanted prejudiced thoughts, remarks or actions from others, you can avoid them and just do breathing exercises with the palms on the knees.

Mental Preparation:

1. Clear your mind of all negativity.
2. Give gratitude for everything that is going on.
3. Relax from toe to head to toe.
4. Close your eyes.
5. Draw your attention inward.

Ideally, these breathing exercises should be practiced twice a day - once in the morning and once in the evening before consciously going to sleep. They should also be done after a yoga session and before the meditation session. The entire process should take ten minutes:

1. Complete breath with holds: 6 cycles: 2 minutes
2. Complete breath with locks: 6 cycles: 2 minutes
3. Alternate nostril breathing: 6 cycles: 4 minutes
4. Core massaging breathing: 12 breaths: 1 minute
5. Relaxed silk breath: 1 minute

Counting: Growing up in India (home of yoga), I was taught to count on the fingers of both hands. Each finger is divided into three segments as you can see by the lines on the palmer surface of the fingers. The thumb is divided into two, but we use the lower section as one, making it also worth three. For the start of counting, we touch the base of the little finger lightly with the thumb of the same hand and leave it there. When we move to the second count, the tip of the thumb is advanced to the middle of the little finger. During count #3, it goes to the top of the little finger and count #4, it goes to the bottom of the ring finger – and so on. This way your mind can count the seconds and not the cycles. When we reach #13, the tip of the index finger is placed on the base of the thumb. With #14, it moves to the middle of the thumb and #15 to the top. #16 will start in the left hand, with the tip of the left thumb touching the base of the left little finger – and so on. So, each hand can count to 15 – and both hands up to 30. During the breathing cycles, you will not go beyond 9. During breathing through both nostrils, each count (each cycle) starts with inspiration. During the alternate nostril breathing, the counts (cycles) start with each inspiration from the left nostril.

Complete breath:

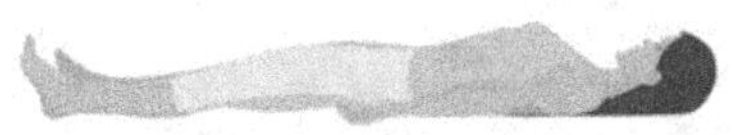

Lie down face up in the *savasana* pose. Place both hands palm down on either side of the belly button with the tips of the middle fingers touching gently. The entire inhalation and the entire exhalation is divided into three sections each - without a specific demarcation. We inhale first into the lower lungs (diaphragm), then into the middle lungs (intercostal muscles) and finally into the upper lung (clavicular muscles) in one smooth continuous action. After a normal pause. we exhale in the reverse direction - first start exhaling from the upper lung, then the middle lung and finally the lower lung. Now inhale, but first fill your lower lung - the belly should move up and the tips of the fingers should separate. The continuing inhalation into the middle lung will result in an expansion of the chest cavity while the final segment - inhalation into the upper lobes will make the collar bone and shoulders rise. After a normal pause. exhalation is done in a controlled but reverse manner - first exhale from the top, then the middle and finally the lower part of the lung. The latter will result in the stomach being sucked in and the middle fingers coming in opposition again. Breathing is done through both nostrils only and the smooth soft process is not accompanied by any sounds or other bodily movements. Inspiration is 5 seconds and expiration is slightly longer - maybe 7-10 seconds. There is a normal pause both at the end of inspiration and the end of expiration. Practice complete breaths 10 times daily whenever you lie down - this not only trains your respiratory muscles to execute the cycle smoothly, it improves your lung capacity, improves the exchange of oxygen and carbon dioxide property of the body, but more importantly, resets over months the medullary pacemaker center, so that your resting and unconscious breathing rate slows down. Remember, during complete breathing, we are executing only 6 or so breaths per minute.

1. Complete breath with holds:

Breathing is done through both nostrils. Always breathe in and out of the nostrils. The sequence is as follows:

Inhalation: 5 seconds
Inspiratory hold: 5 seconds
Expiration: 5 seconds
Expiratory hold: 5 seconds.

Do not follow the count rigidly - if your breath is not complete - either inspiration or expiration, extend or readjust your time accordingly. Normally you may require more time for complete exhalation. The ratio is roughly 1:1:1:1 starting with inspiration. Do this exercise for 6 cycles (2 minutes). Follow up with the complete breath with locks.

2. Complete breath with locks:

A lock in this case involves the pelvic muscles controlling defecation and urination (and also the pelvic sexual organs). There are two locks, which in this exercise are done simultaneously. These are:

- **Mooladhara lock or root lock**: Squeeze the muscles around your anus as you would during defecation or when attempting to stop a fart or defecation. At the same time the muscles of the pelvis are squeezed as you would when you are trying to stop a stream of urination. Both rectal and urinary locks are often done simultaneously in nature. In the root lock, we initiate these two locks together as one lock.

- **Abdominal lock:** This lock squeezes the external and internal muscles of the abdomen associated with breathing. By squeezing the front wall of the belly in (try to pull your belly button backwards to touch your spine).

This exercise is done as the previous exercise except during the expiratory hold, an expiratory lock involving the root and abdominal lock are initiated at the beginning and let go at the end, just before inspiration:

Inhalation: 5 seconds
Inspiratory hold: 5 seconds
Expiration: 5 seconds
Expiratory lock: 5 seconds
Inspiration again
The total cycle takes 20 seconds and you should do 6 cycles (2 minutes) – these timings are approximate.

3. Alternate nostril breathing:

The yogis believe that breathing through the right nostril (sun energy) heats the body and increases catabolism while breathing from the left nostril (moon energy) cools the body and increases anabolism. The aim is to balance the two. The body does so by balancing the sympathetic (flight or fight) system and the opposing parasympathetic system (rest and digest). First close the right nostril with the fleshy tip of the right thumb. Breathe in gently from the left nostril for five seconds. Now with the thumb still on the right nostril, using the same hand, close the left nostril with the ring and little finger. Hold the breath for five seconds. Now let go the thumb while keeping the left nostril closed. Breathe out smoothly over five seconds. Close both nostrils again. Hold for

5 seconds. Now open the right nostril and breathe in from the right nostril for 5 seconds. Close the right nostril again with the right thumb and hold the breath in for 5 seconds. Letting go the little and ring finger, open the left nostril and breathe out for 5 seconds. Close both nostrils and do not breathe for 5 seconds. This is one breath cycle (40 seconds). Restart breathing in from the left nostril to continue the next cycle. Do this for 6 cycles (4 minutes). Remember the ratios starting with left nostril inspiration are as follows 1: 1: 1: 1: 1: 1: 1:1 for the one complete cycle. You can vary the ratio (especially expiration may require more time) according to your convenience. Always initiate this breathing from the left nostril – this will potentiate the good parasympathetic activity and decrease the sympathetic activity - in most millennials, the sympathetic activity is very high.

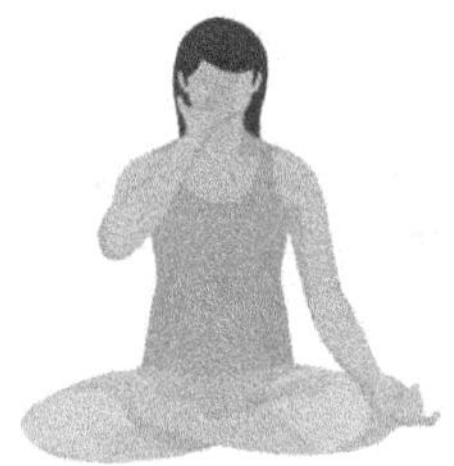

4. **Core massaging breath:**

This is essential to exercise the muscles of respiration and massage the internal organs of the chest and belly. It also massages the organs sheltered in the pelvic area. Take a sudden short and forceful inspiration followed by a normal natural recoil. You should feel the belly bulging out and the chest moving upwards during this forced inspiration. The expiration should be passive and natural. Follow this up with a sudden, short and forceful inspiration again followed by a normal unassisted recoil. This whole inhalation/expiration cycle should take 3-4 seconds. During inspiration you are exercising both the diaphragm and other accessary muscles. Do this for 1 minute.

5. Relaxed silk breath:

Finish off your breathing exercises with calm both nostril breathing in and out without any count. Just concentrate on feeling the silky breath coming in and out of the nostrils. Relax in this breathing mode for one minute, before initiating meditation.

Breathing exercises will bring fresh 'prana' every day and renew your body from inside out.

"Regulate the breathing, and thereby control the mind."

B.K.S. Iyengar

d. Meditation (dhayana)

"Meditation brings wisdom; lack of meditation leaves ignorance. Know well what leads you forward and what holds you back, and choose the path that leads to wisdom."

Buddha

You do not want to be in a mental prison. There is considerable emotional instability in life. You are constantly bombarded with undesirable situations. These troublesome incidents generate thought processes that continue to circulate throughout your brain's neuronal connections, causing irreparable harm – by imbedding the negative experiences as inevitable future happenings, by strengthening erroneous circuits to these stored memories, by erasing positive circuits to better mental destinations, and finally, by preventing the brain to rest and repair. The negative processes do not only continue during conscious thinking, but continue as damaging noises in the subconscious - even during sleep. They often become solidly entrenched in your brain – probably during REM sleep.

These destructive emotions include:

1. Abuse: I have been abused all my life.

2. Alienation: I have been alienated - nobody likes me.

3. Anger: I am constantly misunderstood and being wronged. I am angry at myself and everyone else.

4. Anxiety: My future remains uncertain – personally, socially and economically, I am scared of 'bad things' that may happen in my future.

5. Apathy - I am worthless. Nothing is worth anything anymore. Why even try doing something?

6. Bitterness: I am bitter about a lot of things.

7. Depression: I feel hopeless and helpless.

8. Ego: I am the best. I know it all.

9. Fear: I fear everything – including myself and the almighty.

10. Frustration: I am not getting what I want.

11. Greed: I need more. I deserve more.

12. Grief: I will continue to lose things with age – my family, my assets, my health.

13. Guilt: Where did I go wrong? I should have done better in life.

14. Hate: I hate everything and everybody.

15. Humiliation/Shame: I am not as good as I should be.

16. Jealousy: I will become more important or rich than the other person.

17. Loneliness: Nobody understands me. I have nobody who trusts me or loves me.

18. Loss: I do not want to lose what I have.

19. Pessimism: I will never amount to anything now. There is no future for me.

20. Sadness: I am sad. I feel like crying. I am depressed.

21. Self-doubt: Maybe I do not know what to do. I am going to be a failure.

22. Separation: I miss my family and friends.

23. Suspicion: I cannot trust anyone.

24. Victimization: I am not able to succeed because of my race,

religion or ethnicity or some other bias.

And there are many more. Unfortunately, everyone around you may be subject to similar emotions. It is how they handle it makes a difference. Some shrug them off and continue forward with their lives. Some hold on to them and let them grow like cancer – destroying their life. Some seek professional help. And some may just want a sympathetic ear – to vent their shortcomings. How you respond to these unwanted situations in your life will decide your emotional future – one of continued distress or one of serenity. Yoga will help you in clearing your flawed thinking and erroneous response to these - and allow you to take a positive approach. It will help you become somewhat 'emotion' proof. Meditation will help.

"God grant me the serenity
To accept the things I cannot change;
Courage to change the things I can;
And wisdom to know the difference."

Reinhold Neibuhr (1892-1971)

Disturbed emotions can also negatively impact spirituality.

"Just as a candle cannot burn without fire, men cannot live without a spiritual life."

Buddha

Detrimental emotional factors (both external and internal) also strip away the protective layer of spirituality. As the processes continue, the inner core of spirituality is also leached away - leaving you significantly spiritually depleted. You become distressed and helpless, often questioning:

1. Why me?
2. Is there enough time for me to reverse my life process for the better?
3. Is there a higher power?

Without spirituality, you do not appreciate life (who am I?), the real life in life (what am I here for?), the now in life (past and future are just embedded in the now). You do not appreciate why you have things and why you do not. You do not recognize the underlying reason why you do things and why you do not. You do not understand why things happen and why they do not. You have false notions about life and you get either over-elated or extremely frustrated. This robs you of the very essence of life - to have a peaceful and happy journey. A grateful spirit will:

- Help you appreciate life.
- Help you enjoy the life in life.
- Help you acknowledge with thanks what you have.
- Help you appreciate every moment as being special – especially the now in time.
- Help you recognize that you are powerless over certain events - and this is ok.
- Help you accept and positively learn from your mistakes and failures.
- Help you be content with what we are.
- Help you get closer to our creator - the omnipotent and omnipresent universal source.

"Every human being's essential nature is perfect and faultless, but after years of immersion in the world, we easily forget our roots and take on a counterfeit nature."

Lao- Tzu

Yogic meditation will help you become more positive and stop and reverse this spiritual depletion. You will discover that meditation is calming to the brain and helps curtail and slow down the negative thoughts racing in an uncontrolled manner through your brain. Affirmative meditation will help erase these negative circuits and through neuro-plasticity, create newer positive circuits that will bring you peace and happiness.

Meditation should follow the asanas and prayanamas. You have achieved calmness of the body through asanas and calmness of the breath through pranayamas. Meditation will help you achieve stillness of the mind. Ideally stay in the same position and same environment following the breathing exercises.

Meditation poses

Meditation is facilitated if done in the following poses: (These have also been described in the asanas section)

1. **Easy Pose** *(Sukhasana)*

1.   Breathing normally, lower your torso, place both hands on the floor, sit down on your buttocks and straighten out the legs in front of you. The arms are resting along your sides.
2.   Sit up straight. (This is the *dandasana* pose)
3.   Cross your legs in front of you and fold them near your torso.
4.   With the knees wide apart, tuck your feet beneath the opposite knee. Either shin can be on top – it is good to alternate on different days. The position should be easy and relaxed.
5.   Place your palms on the knees, facing down or up, and without any tension. Adopt a mudra that you feel comfortable with. (breathing mudras described after these poses)
6.   Hold this pose. Gaze is front infinity. Breathe normally.

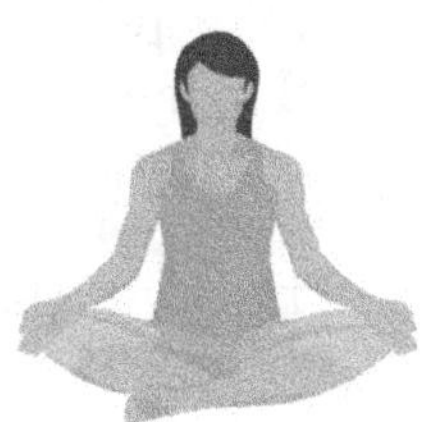

2. **Corpse Pose** *(savasana)*

1.   Lie down on the floor with face up. The entire body should be aligned and relaxed.

2.   Bring the arms by the sides and the hands on the knees with the palms facing up.
3.   The legs normally rotate out with the toes facing up and away from each other.
4.   Make sure you are in a 'neutral' position with no tension.
5.   Breathe nice and easy through the nostrils.

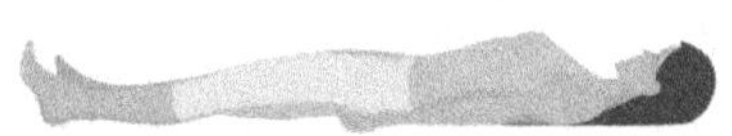

Meditation can also be done in the following poses:

3. **Perfect pose** *(siddhasan)*

1. Breathing normally, lower your torso, place both hands on the floor, sit down on your buttocks and straighten out the legs in front of you.
2. Sit up straight. (*dandasana* pose)
3. Now bending your left knee slide the left heel towards the groin. Leave the heel in this position touching your groin.
4. Bend the right knee and bring the right ankle over the left ankle, resting it near your pubic bone (the central bone above your groin)
5. Rest your hands on the knees and adopt a meditation

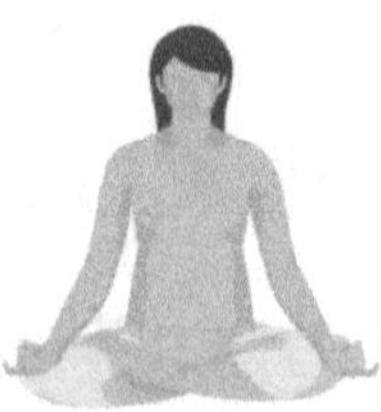

mudra.

4. **Hero pose** *(Virasana)*

1.   From the *tadasana* pose, inhaling, bend forward, lower your body and place your knees on the floor. The legs go backwards perpendicular to the thighs but parallel to each other on the floor. Your torso and head are straight up, in line with the thighs.
2.   Place your hands on the thighs. Sit back with your buttocks in between the two legs. Your position should be snug with the outer thighs in contact with your inner calves.
4.   Chest should be straight up with the face looking forward. Gaze would be front infinity.
5.   Hold position. Breathe normally. If you are unable to sit on the floor, sit on a folded blanket placed in between your thighs/feet.
6.   Adopt a hand mudra according to your preference.

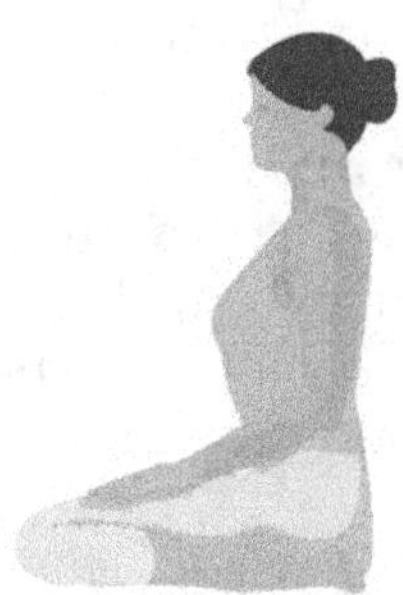

Meditation Mudras:

Meditation is often accompanied by hand gestures that aid in attaining the silence of the mind that we are trying to achieve. The two mudras that I find are conducive to this are:

1. **Anjali Mudra**: Use this to start and end your meditation. In this pose, also called the prayer pose, bring both palms together in the middle of the chest, softly but firmly pressing against each other. The thumbs are touching the breast bone while the finger tips are facing upwards.

2. **Dhyani Mudra**: After initiating meditation with the anjali mudra, change your hands into this mudra. Place your left hand on top of your right hand, both open flat with the palms facing up. The hands are placed on the lap with both little fingers towards the belly. The tips of the thumbs are made to touch each other forming an oval in the front. At the end of meditation, transit into the Anjali mudra again momentarily before retiring or getting up.

A. Meditations:

Find a quiet period or a quiet place (outdoors) try the following:

1. **Silk breath meditation**: Monitor your breath coming in and out of your nostrils and gently caressing them. Your thoughts should be completely devoted to following the breath. Mentally counting the time slowly – one Mississippi (one second) onwards – both during inspiration (say 3 seconds) and expiration (3-4 seconds), helps prevent the mind from wandering.

3. **Mantra meditation**: In this, repeat a mantra, ideally as a whisper or if not possible - in the mind. The Hindus like to use Aum. A phrase can be picked up from the bible or other religious texts and repeated. Verbalization appears to benefit with the resultant vibrations produced.

4. **Thoughtless meditation**: This is my favorite but may take some time to learn. You divert your attention towards your third eye, inside the head behind the eyebrows. Now you think of nothing - try to be thoughtless. If thoughts occur, remove them and again become thoughtless. Although it sounds impossible, it is do-able. And the brain truly becomes silent. You reap all the benefits of meditation.

Do meditation, after the breathing session. If you fall off into a sleep - fine. Meditation can also be done independently - before any preceding asanas or breathing exercises. Make sure the place, pose and conditions are kept as close to as possible to those listed under yoga and pranayama.

Besides the meditative practices described above, it is important that you understand and learn two other meditation techniques based on developing happiness and positivity. You can use these at anytime and anywhere. Resorting to these two techniques (positive visualization and positive affirmations) should be spontaneous, when anticipating or facing a disturbing situation – you will find immediate inner solace - and the final results of the undesired event will be better. These can be done even if just thinking of a negative event in the past or a potentially negative event in the future. Close your eyes and do these meditations, even if it is for a few seconds. Learning to do them with your eyes open will help you practice them in situations where you cannot close your eyes.

B. MEDITATIVE VISUALIZATION

This is important for removing some of the negativity stemming from loneliness and hardships encountered during life. Closing your eyes and imagining yourself in your favorite experienced place, position or among your favorite people or things is extremely beneficial to your underlying brain wiring:

1. It prevents negative thoughts from occurring, thereby not strengthening those storage neurons and the negative pathways, at least during the positive visualization. On the flip side, it helps fortify the positive stores in the brain and their connections - thereby raising baseline hope and happiness, though at a subconscious level.

2. It removes negative external distractions during the period of positive visualization - and allows you to live in the 'now'. For example, while in the shower think of being on a beach or a spa and taking a shower under luxurious natural or man-made environment. You will enjoy your shower more and even clean yourself better. Even a simple shower will leave you mentally invigorated. You will actually feel gratitude for the shower - a good thing.

3. Positive visualization prior to sleep may transfer your negative dreams into positive happy ones. You will sleep better and wake up happier.

4.Positive visualizations translate into positive intent - it will help you look forward to a better future on discharge.

"Feelings come and go like clouds in a windy sky. Conscious breathing is my anchor."

Thich Nhat Hanh

C. MEDITATIVE AFFIRMATIONS *and* GRATITUDE

"We have been taught to believe that negative equals realistic and positive equals unrealistic."

Susan Jeffers

The emotional upheavals of everyday life slowly harms you. In order to build a barrier to these, and also rewrite your own negative neuronal biology, practice positive affirmations in a meditative state - closed eyes and in a quiet place. This can be done outside your yoga practice or added to it.

Your thoughts at any time should be positive and uplifting. Repeat these affirmations whenever you can and as often as you can:

1. I am a good person.
2. I am a healthy person.
3. I am a loving person.
4. I am a caring person.
5. I am a capable person.
6. I am loved person.
7. I am an honest person.
8. I am full of vitality.
9. I am a happy person.
10. I am one with the Source.

Repeat these affirmations during meditation periods. Affirmations result in activation of areas of the brain that are responsible for self-processing (medial prefrontal cortex + posterior cingulate cortex [1,2] and reward/valuation (ventral striatum + ventral medial prefrontal cortex)[3]. Repeating positive affirmations over a period of time, will rewire the brain and change the electrical routes to the more positive centers in the brain – a positive neuroplasticity. Positivity results in the brain ordered production of serotonin and a decrease in cortisol – changes that produce feelings of happiness. Other beneficial hormones released with positivity - and happiness include dopamine, oxytocin, and endorphins[4].

"Those who have the ability to be grateful are the ones who have the ability to achieve greatness."

Steve Maraboli

And also, be thankful, especially before going to sleep:

1. I am thankful for continuing my soul's journey in this body – allowing me to experience being a human.
2. I am thankful for being able to live this experience and learn from it.
3. I am thankful for everything I have received during this journey.
4. I am thankful for joys spent during good times and the lessons learnt from adversity.
5. I am thankful for the mastering the ability to live in the present - not regretting the past or fretting about the future.
6. I am at peace - accepting serenely what I cannot change.
7. I am thankful to my spirit for keeping me energized.
8. I am thankful to the Universal Creator for providing me with this energy and keeping my soul's journey on its course.

"The mountains, I become part of it
The herb, the fir tree, I become a part of it
The morning mist, the clouds, the gathering waters
I become part of it
The wilderness, the dew drop, the pollen...
I become a part of it."

Navajo Chant

8.Sequence II

a. Asanas (Sequence II – additions)

Once you feel comfortable with the above routine, and have it kind of memorized, you may want to incorporate 30 more asanas – interspersed in the first routine. These thirty are described below. The flow should still be continuous and fluid, despite the new additions.

STANDING POSES

1. Mountain Pose
2. Upward Salute

2a. Swaying Tree Pose Right side *(Tiryaka tadasana)*

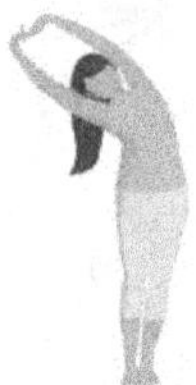

2b. Swaying Tree Pose Left side *(Tiryaka tadasana)*

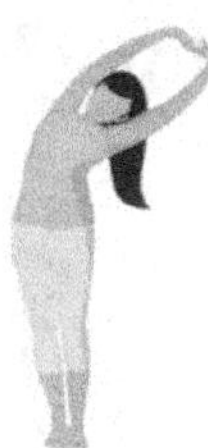

2c. Tree Pose Right *(Vrikshasana)*

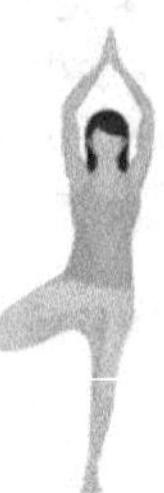

2d. Tree Pose Right *(Vrikshasana)*

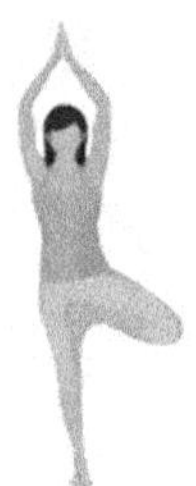

3.Standing half forward bend

3a. Extended Hand-To-Big-Toe Pose Right leg up *(Utthita Hasta Padangusthasana)*

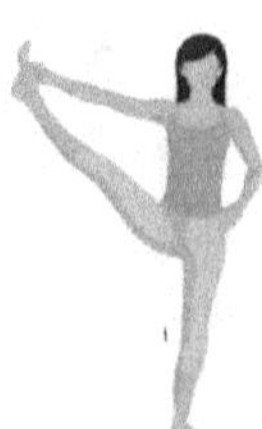

3b. Extended Hand-To-Big-Toe Pose Left leg up
(Utthita Hasta Padangusthasana)

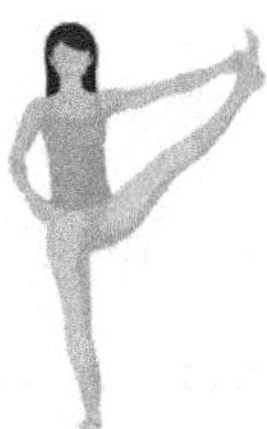

4. Modified Mountain Pose
5. Crescent Moon in Mountain Pose
6. Deep Forward Bend
7. Right Leg Forward Bend Both Hands
8. Left Leg Forward Bend Both Hands
9. Wide Legged Mountain Pose
10. Both Hands to Right Big Toe Pose; With left hand up / revolve to right hand up
11. Both Hands to Left Big Toe Pose; With right hand up / revolve to left hand up
12. Crescent Moon in Wide Legged Mountain Pose
13. Forward Bend with palms on floor

13a: **Wide-Legged Standing Forward Fold**
(Prasarita Padottanasana)

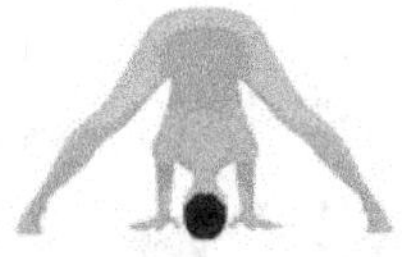

14. Right Side Bend in Wide Legged Mountain Pose

14a: **Balancing star *(Utthita Ardha Chandrasana)***

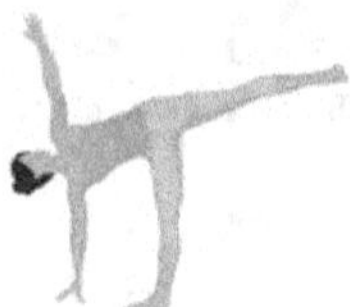

15.Left Side Bend in Wide Legged Mountain Pose

15a: **Balancing star *(Utthita Ardha Chandrasana)***

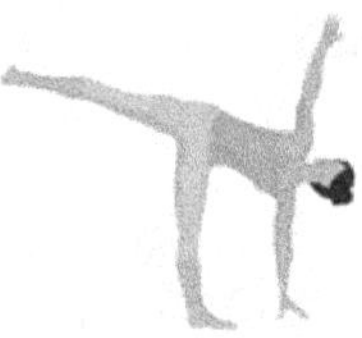

16.   Warrior I: Right Foot Forward - Right Knee Bent
17.   Forward High Lunge in Warrior I Right Foot Forward - Right Knee Bent
18.   Reverse Warrior with Right Foot Forward - Right Knee Bent

18a. **Extended Side Angle Pose Right leg bent *(Utthita Parsvakonasana)***

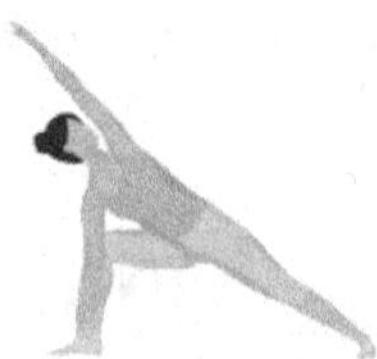

18b. **Revolved Side Angle Pose Right leg bent *(Parivrtta Parsvakonasana)***

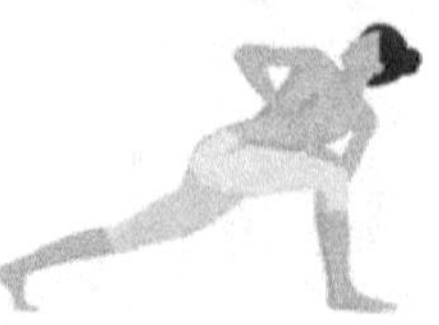

19. Warrior I: Left Foot Forward - Left Knee Bent
20. Forward High Lunge in Warrior I: Left Foot Forward - Left Knee Bent
21. Reverse Warrior with Left Foot Forward

21a. Extended Side Angle Pose Left leg bent (*Utthita Parsvakonasana*)

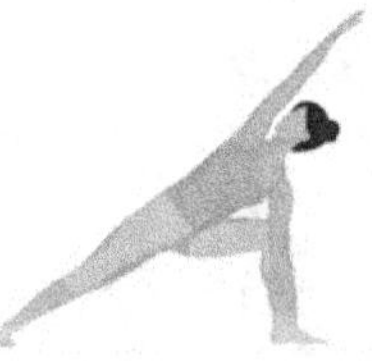

21b. Revolved Side Angle Pose Left leg bent (*Parivrtta Parsvakonasana*)

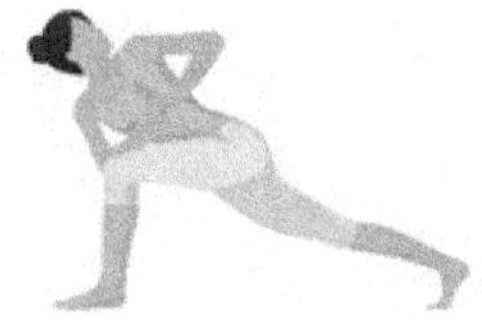

22. Warrior II with Right Knee Bent - Twist Right and hold and then Left
23. Warrior II with Left Knee Bent - Twist Left and hold and then Right
24. Standing Chair

KNEELING/SITTING POSES:

25. Garland
26. Hero Pose

26a: **Half Spinal Twist Pose – Twist right side (*Vakrasana*)**

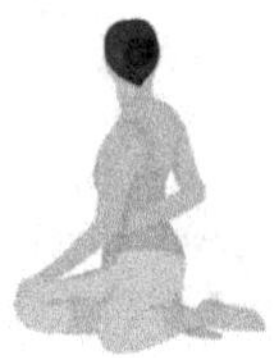

26b: **Half Spinal Twist Pose – Twist left side (*Vakrasana*)**

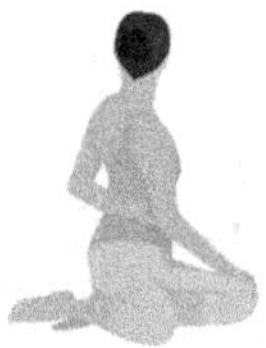

27. Easy Pose
28. Butterfly
29. Staff Pose
30. Half Bound Forward Bend - Right Leg Straight
31. Half Bound Forward Bend - Left Leg Straight

31a: **Revolved Head to Knee Pose Right side (*Parivrtta Janu Sirsasana*)**

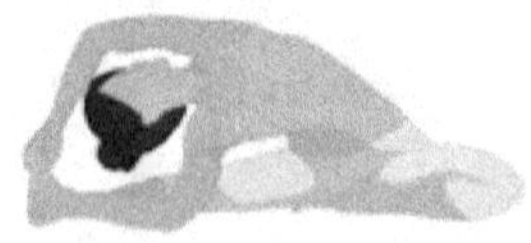

**31b: Revolved Head to Knee Pose Left side
(*Parivrtta Janu Sirsasana*)**

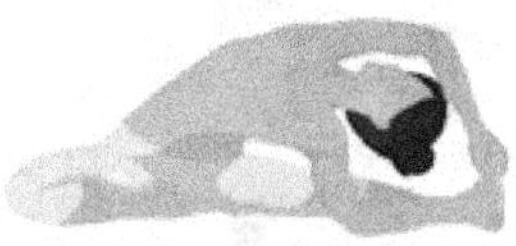

32. Thunderbolt Pose
33. Crescent Moon in Hero Pose
34. Child Pose
35. Extended Puppy Pose
36. Standing Thunderbolt

36a: Camel Pose (*Ustrasana*)

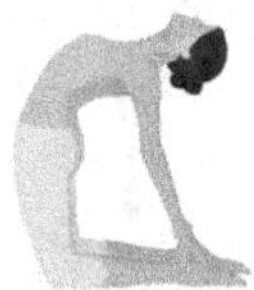

37. Gate Latch: Right Leg Extended
38. Gate Latch: Left Leg Extended
39. Downward Facing Dog
40. Low Lunge: Lizard: Right Knee Front and Bent

**40a: Modified low lung Right Knee Front and Bent
(*Modified Anjaneyasana*)**

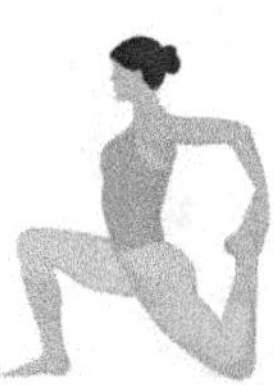

41.   Low Lunge: Lizard: Left Knee Front and Bent

41a. Modified low lung Left Knee Front and Bent *(Modified Anjaneyasana)*

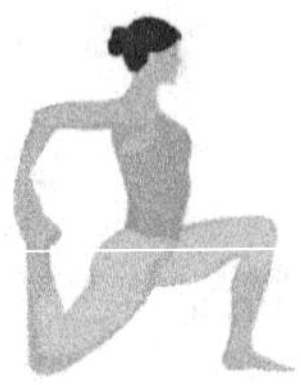

41b. Reverse Corpse Pose *(Advasana)*

LYING FACE DOWN POSES

42.   Sphynx

42a. Dolphin Pose *(Ardha Pincha Mayurasana)*

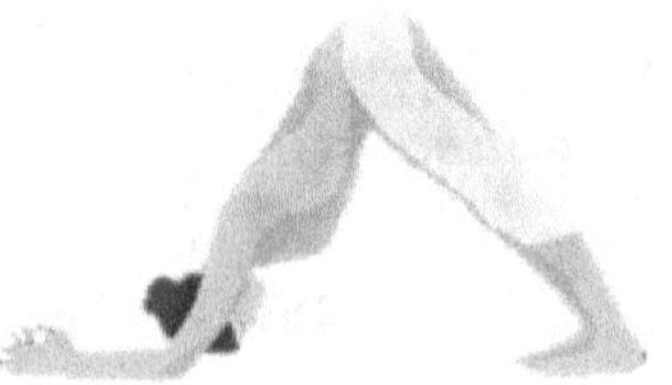

43.   Dolphin Plank
44.   Cobra
45.   Upward Facing Dog
46.   Downward Facing Plank

46a. Four Limbed Staff Pose *(Chaturanga Dandasana)*

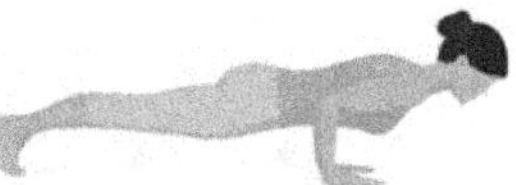

46b. Cat Pose *(Marjaiasana)*

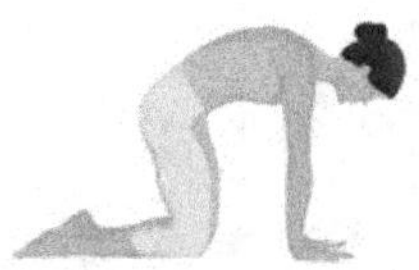

46c. Cow Pose *(Bitilasana)*

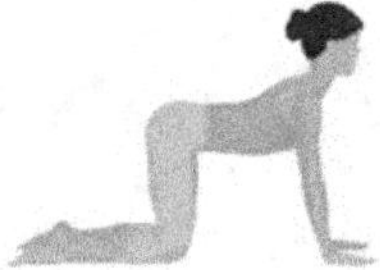

47. Locust
48. Bow
49. Reclining Buddha: Right Side

49a. Reclining Buddha Right side with Left leg up

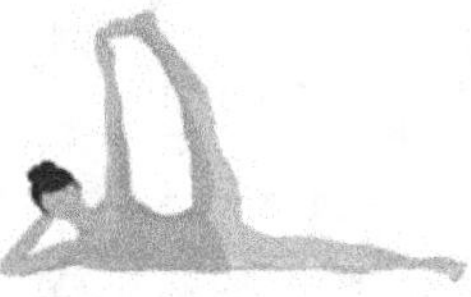

50. Side Plank: Right Side
51. Reclining Buddha: Left Side

51a. Reclining Buddha Left side with Right leg up

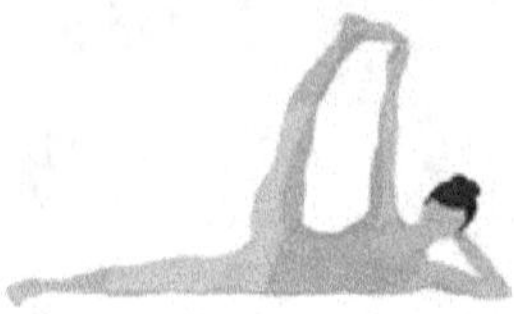

52. Side Plank: Left Side

LYING FACE UP POSES

53. Corpse Pose
54. Boat - Full Boat

54a. Fish Pose *(Matsyasana)*

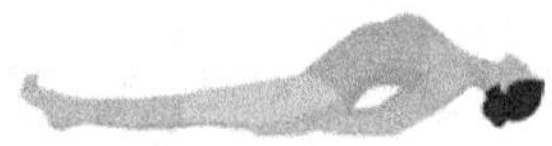

55. Happy Baby Pose
56. Wind Relief Pose
57. Bridge Pose
58. Upward Plank

58a. Reclining Bound Angle Pose *(Supta Baddha Konasana)*

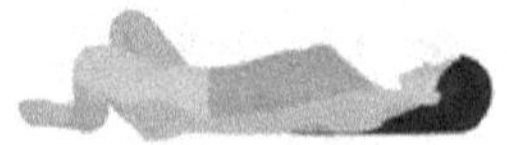

59. Supine Spinal Twist Right Side
60. Supine Spinal Twist Left Side

60a. **Shoulder Stand** *(Salamba Sarvangasana)*

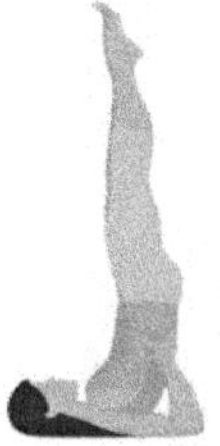

Final: Corpse pose to supine stretch and back to corpse pose.

DETAILED NEW POSES FOR THE SEQUENCE II

Previous Pose

#2

Tiryaka tadasana

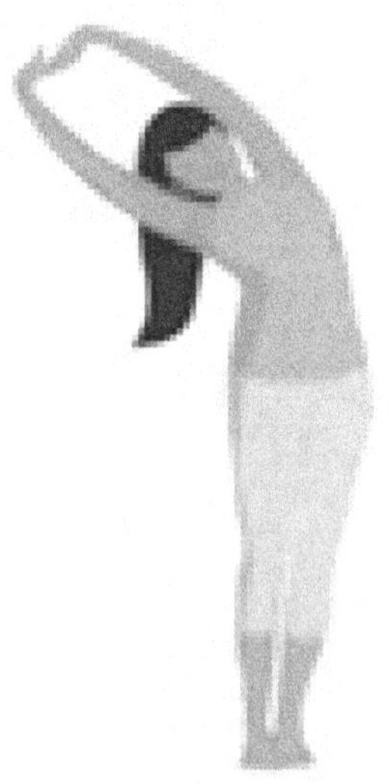

SWAYING TREE POSE (Right side sway)
#2a

2a.SWAYING TREE POSE (Right side sway)

1. Stand in the Mountain Pose.
2. Look straight forward at infinity.
3. Interlock the fingers of both hands in front of the body. The palms are facing the floor.
4. Raise the arms above the head and stretch upwards.
5. Bend from the waist to the right side, keeping the arms stretched.

Breathing:

1. Inhalation on raising the arms over the head.
2. Exhalation during waist bending.
3. Breathe normal during hold.
4. Inhalation on releasing the bend.

Gaze: Front/infinity

Transition pose: Mountain pose

Next pose: Swaying Tree

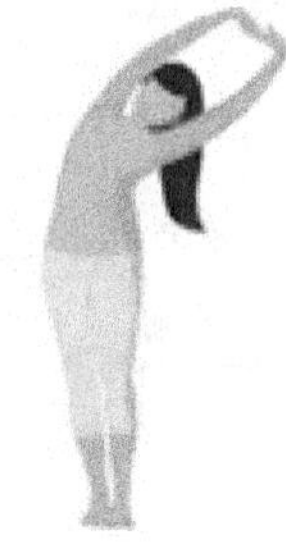

#2b

Previous Pose

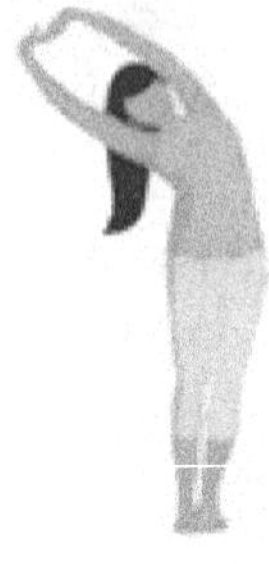

#2a

Tiryaka tadasana

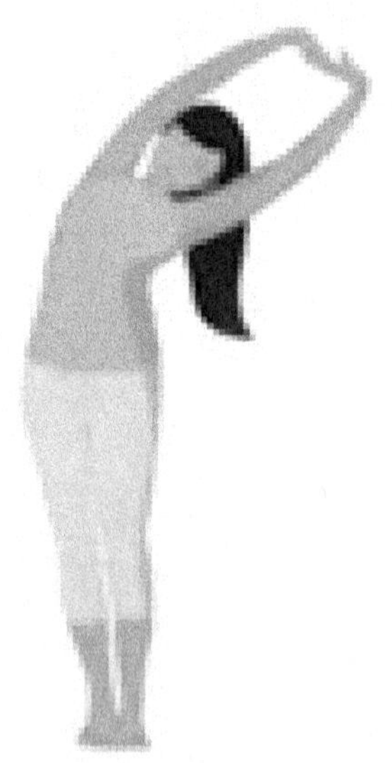

SWAYING TREE POSE
#2b

2b.SWAYING TREE POSE (Left side sway)

1. Start in the Mountain Pose.
2. Look straight forward at infinity.
3. Interlock the fingers of both hands in front of the body. The palms are facing the floor.
4. Raise the arms above the head and stretch upwards.
5. Bend from the waist to the left side, keeping the arms stretched.

Breathing:

1. Inhalation on raising the arms over the head.
2. Exhalation during waist bending.
3. Breathe normal during hold.
4. Inhalation on releasing the bend.

Gaze: Front/infinity

Transition pose: Mountain Pose

Next pose: Tree pose

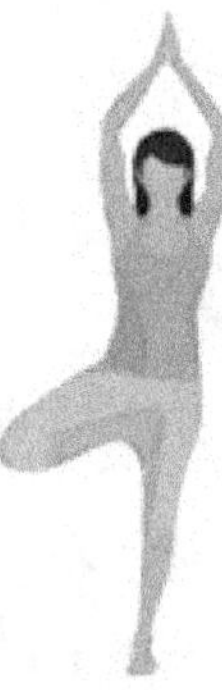

#2c

Previos Pose

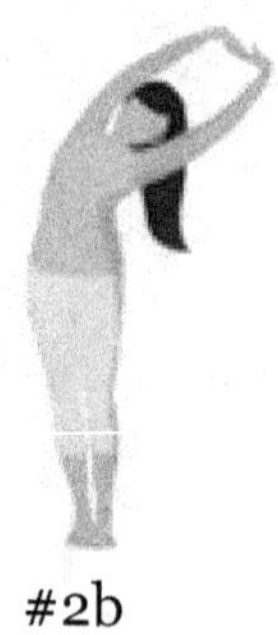

#2b

Vrksasana

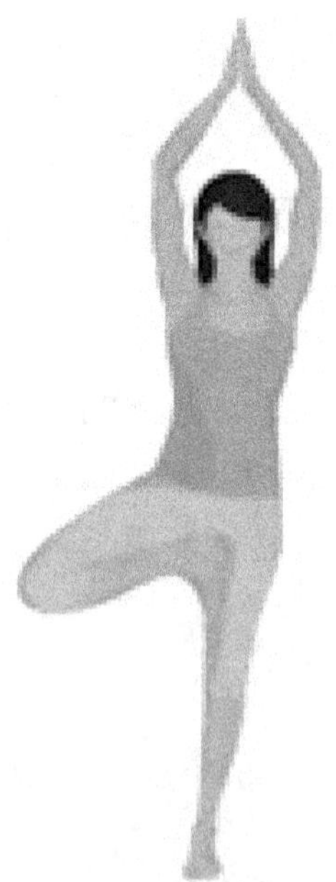

TREE POSE (Right Leg Up)
#2c

2c. TREE POSE (Right Leg Up)

1. From the *Tadasana* – Mountain Pose, shift your weight onto the left leg and bend the right knee. The right knee should be facing the right side and the right heel should be against the left leg.
2. Slowly slide up the right foot up the left leg to the highest point where you can balance safely.
3. Now while inhaling, lift your arms over your head with the palms facing each other and touching.

Breathing:

1. Inhalation on raising the arms.
2. Normal during hold.

Gaze: Front/infinity

Transition pose: Mountain Pose

Next pose: Tree Pose

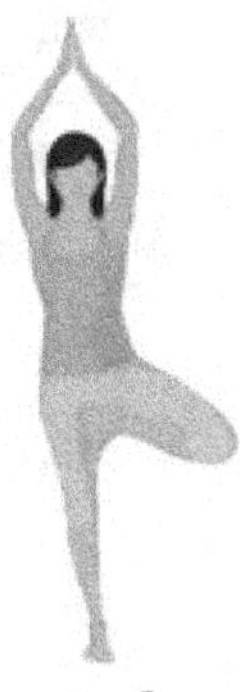

#2d

Previous Pose

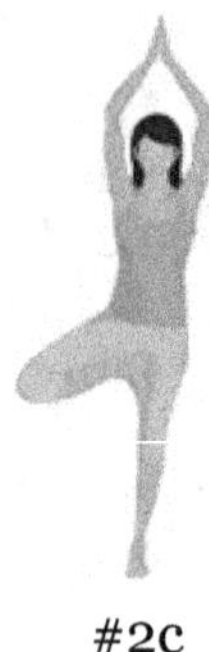

#2c

Vrksasana

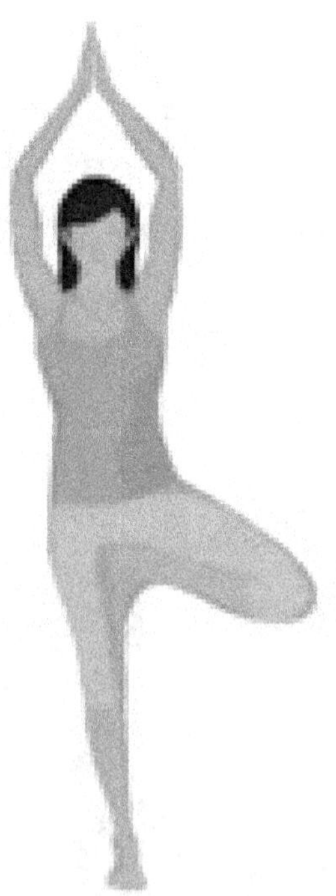

TREE POSE (Left leg up)
#2d

2d. TREE POSE (Left leg up)

1. From the *Tadasana* – Mountain Pose, shift your weight onto the right leg and bend the left knee. The left knee should be facing the left side and the left heel should be against the right leg.
2. Slowly slide up the left foot up the right leg to the highest point where you can balance safely.
3. Now while inhaling, lift your arms over your head with the palms facing each other and touching.

Breathing:

1. Inhalation on raising the arms.
2. Normal during hold.

Gaze: Front/infinity

Transition pose: Mountain pose

Next pose: Half Forward Bend

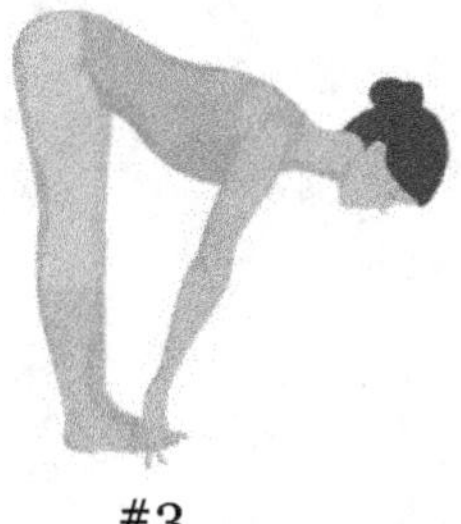

#3

Previous Pose

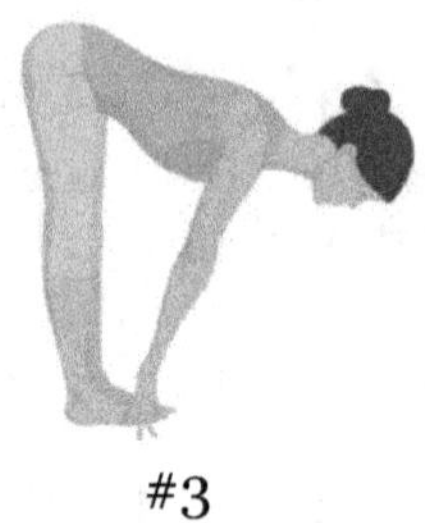

#3

Utthita Hasta Padangusthasana

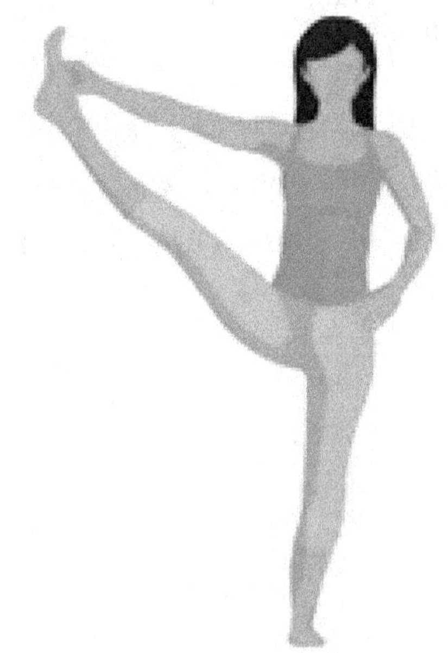

EXTENDED HAND TO BIG TOE POSE (Right leg up)
#3a

3a. EXTENDED HAND TO BIG TOE POSE (Right leg up)

1. Start in the *Tadasana* Pose.
2. Putting your weight on the left leg, slowly bend the right knee and bring the leg up with the knee facing the front.
3. Hold the right ankle with the right hand.
4. Straighten the right leg in front as far as you can without losing balance.
5. Now swing the right hand and right leg to the right side as far as you can.

Breathing:

1. Normal during hold.

Gaze: Front/infinity

Transition pose: Mountain Pose

Next pose: Extended hand to big toe

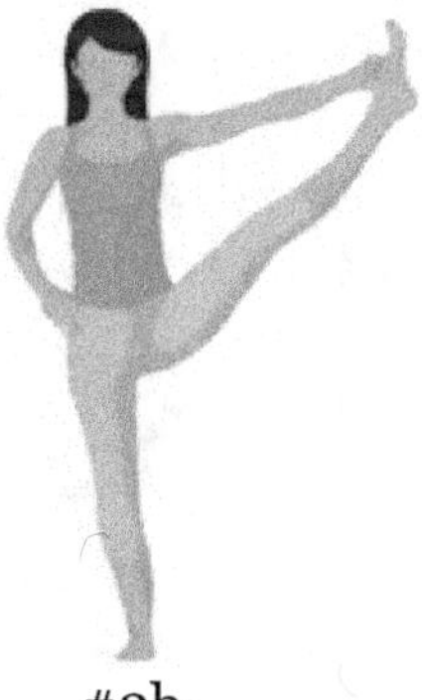

#3b

Previous Pose

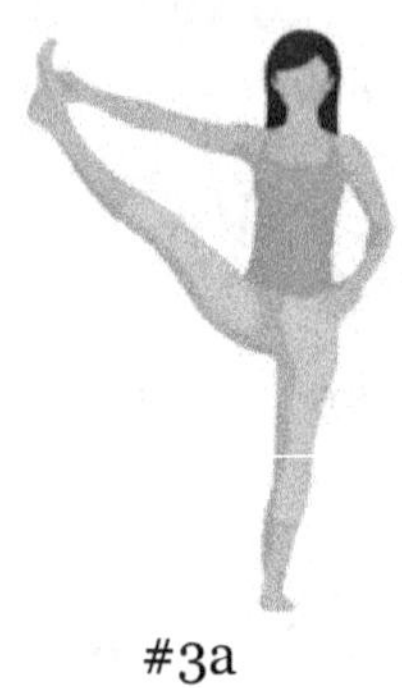

#3a

Utthita Hasta Padangusthasana

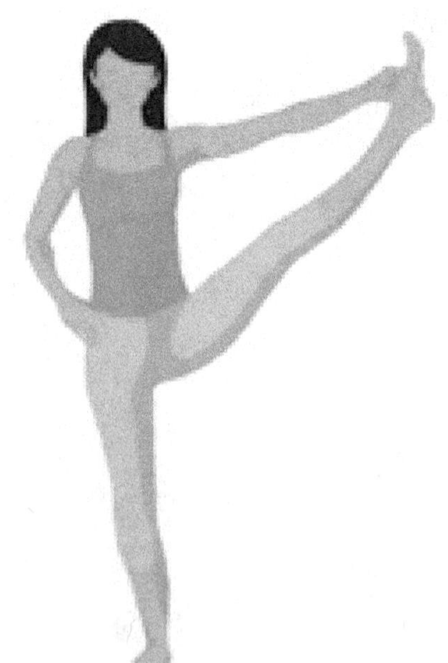

EXTENDED HAND TO BIG TOE POSE (left leg up)
#3b

3b. EXTENDED HAND TO BIG TOE POSE (left leg up)

1.   Start in the *Tadasana* Pose.
2.   Putting your weight on the right leg, slowly bend the left knee and bring the leg up with the knee facing the front.
3.   Hold the left ankle with the left hand.
4.   Straighten the left leg in front as far as you can without losing balance.
5.   Now swing the left hand and left leg to the left side as far as you can.

Breathing:

1.   Normal during hold.

Gaze: Front/infinity

Transition pose: None

Next pose: Modified Mountain

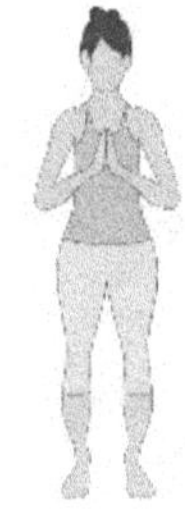

#4

Previous Pose

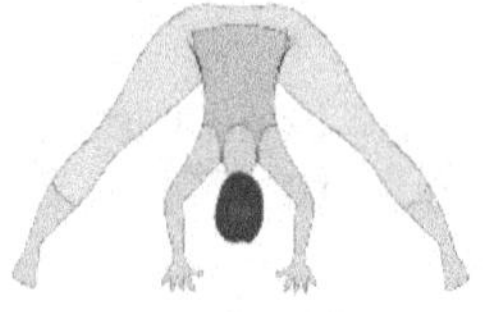

#13

Prasarita Padottanasana

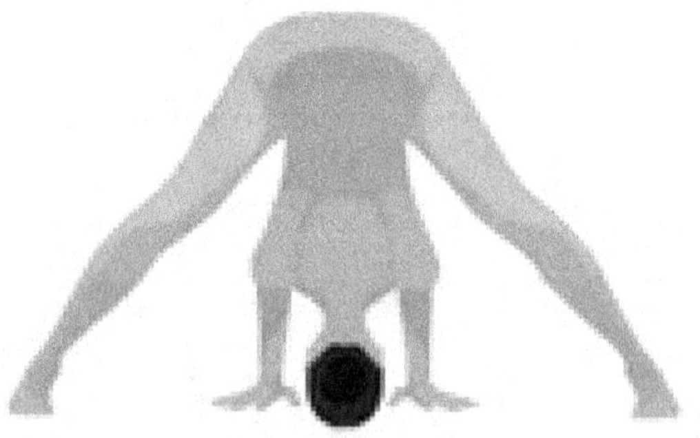

WIDE-LEGGED STANDING FORWARD FOLD
#13a

13a. WIDE-LEGGED STANDING FORWARD FOLD

1. From the wide legged mountain pose, inhaling lengthen your torso upwards. Now exhaling bend forward at the hips and bring both palms of the hands on the floor in front of you, if possible.
2. The hands are now between your legs.
3. Move your hands backwards towards your legs and then bring your head as close to the floor as possible.
4. Ideally your crown of the head should rest on the floor.
5. To come out of the pose, first bring both hands on the hips and then straighten.

Breathing:

1. Exhalation on way down.
2. Normal during hold.

Gaze: Front/infinity or hands

Next Pose: Right sided bend in WLMP

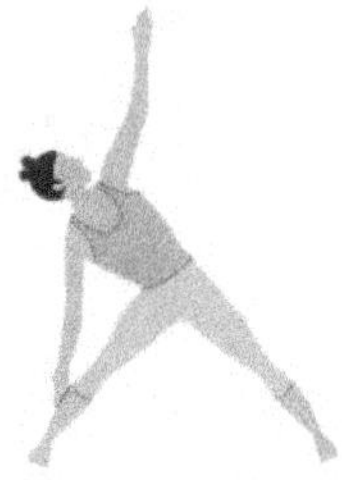

#14

Previous Pose

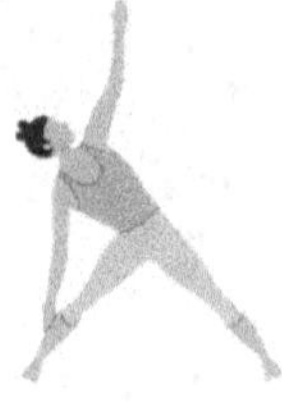

#14

Utthita Ardha Chandrasana

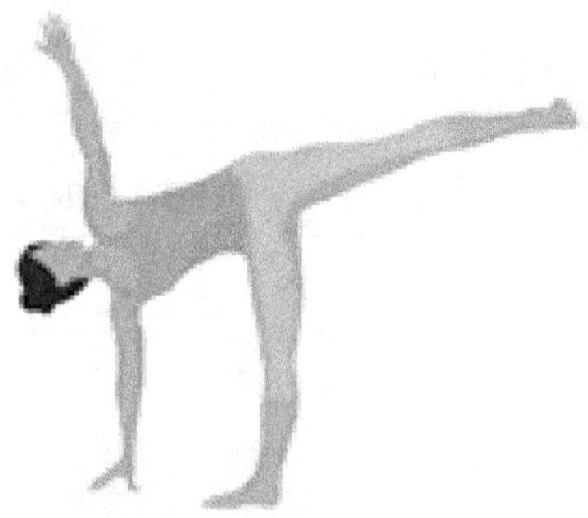

BALANCING STAR (Right leg down)
#14a

14a. **BALANCING STAR (Right leg down)**

1. From the wide legged mountain pose turn your right toes facing right. The left foot remains firm with the toes facing forward. Both heels should be aligned along the same line. Look straight forward.
2. Inhaling spread out your arms to the sides at shoulder level.
3. Exhaling, bend at your waist towards the right, and slide your right hand down along the shin of the right leg to the right ankle.
4. The left arm should be simultaneously raised upwards with the shoulders being aligned on top of each other.
5. From here, walk your right hand away from the right foot with the palm on the floor.
6. At the same time lift your left leg up and try to reach a balance pose.
7. You are now resting on the right hand and right foot.
8. Your gaze should be upwards at the left-hand thumb.

Breathing:

1. Normal during hold.

Gaze: upper hand.

Next pose: Left side bend in WLMP

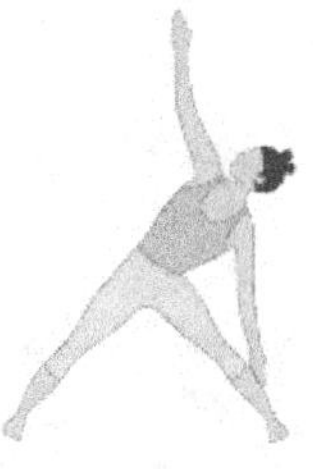

#15

Previous Pose

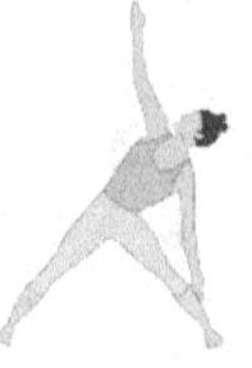

#15

Utthita Ardha Chandrasana

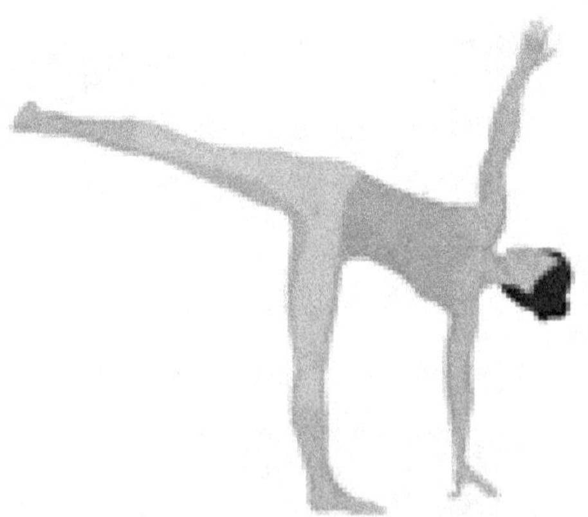

BALANCING STAR (Left leg down)
#15a

15a. BALANCING STAR (Left leg down)

1. From the wide legged mountain pose turn your left toes facing left. The right foot remains firm with the toes facing forward. Both heels should be aligned along the same line. Look straight forward.
2. Inhaling spread out your arms to the sides at shoulder level.
3. Exhaling, bend at your waist towards the left, and slide your left hand down along the shin of the left leg to the left ankle.
4. The right arm should be simultaneously raised upwards with the shoulders being aligned on top of each other.
5. From here, walk your left hand away from the left foot with the palm on the floor.
6. At the same time lift your right leg up and try to reach a balance pose.
7. You are now resting on the left hand and left foot.
8. Your gaze should be upwards at the right-hand thumb.

Breathing:

1. Normal during hold.

Gaze: upper hand.

Next pose: Warrior I Right leg forward

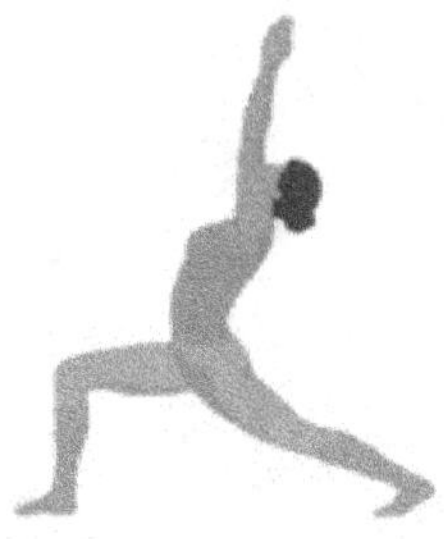

Previous Pose

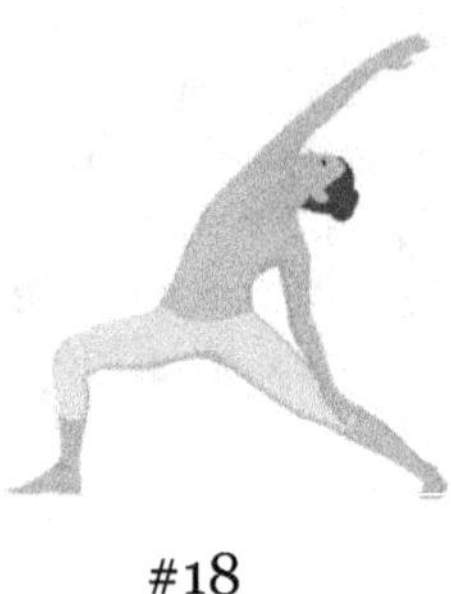

#18

Utthita Parsvakonasana

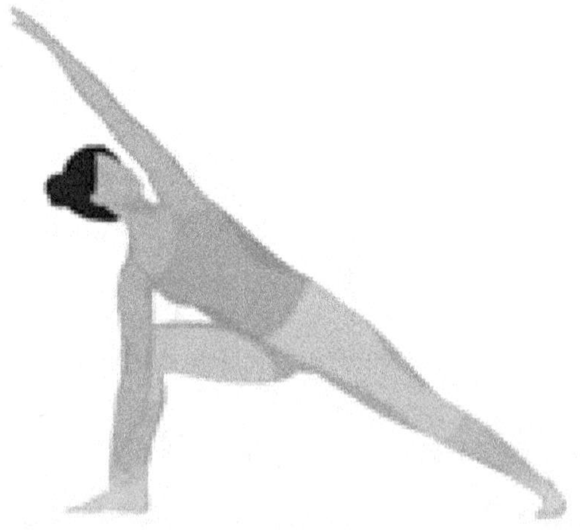

EXTENDED SIDE ANGLE POSE (Right leg bent)
#18a

18a. EXTENDED SIDE ANGLE POSE (Right leg bent)

1. From the mountain pose, spread your legs shoulder or more apart.
2. Turn your right leg and foot outward 90 degrees so your toes point to the right side.
3. Bend your right knee until your right thigh is parallel to the floor. Keep your right knee directly over your right heel.
4. Bending to the right from the waist, bring your right arm in front of the right leg and lower it as far as you can, preferably with the right palm on the floor just in front of the right foot.
5. Now raise and straighten your left arm in the direction of the right toes with your arm touching the left ear.
6. Look upwards while holding this pose.

Breathing:

1. Normal during hold.

Gaze: upwards/infinity

Transition pose: None

Next pose: Revolved side angle pose right leg bent

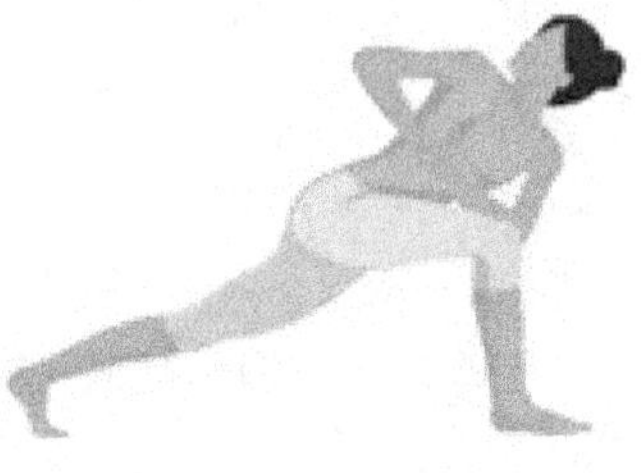

#18b

Previous Pose

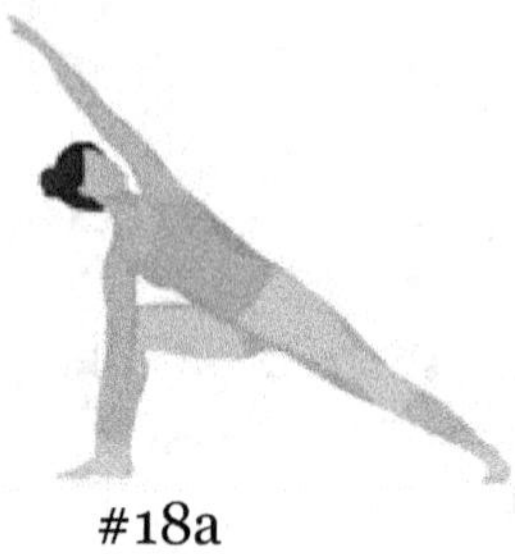

#18a

Parivrtta Parsvakonasana

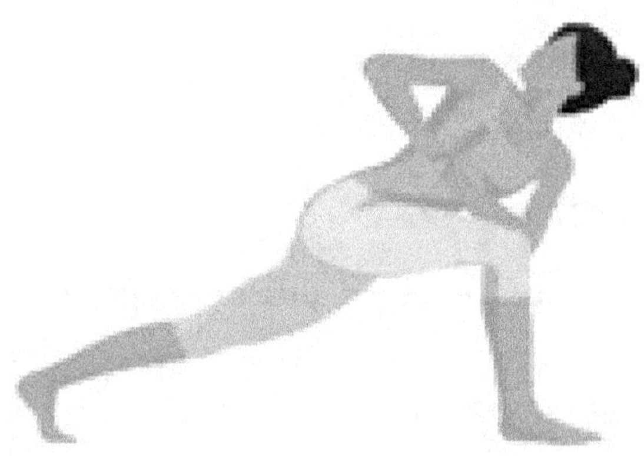

REVOLVED SIDE ANGLE POSE (Right leg bent)
#18b

18b. REVOLVED SIDE ANGLE POSE (Right leg bent)

1   From the mountain pose, spread your legs shoulder or more apart.
2. Turn your right leg and foot outward 90 degrees so your toes point to the right side.
3. Bend your right knee until your right thigh is parallel to the floor. Keep your right knee directly over your right heel.
4. Bending your torso rightwards and downwards, bring your left arm in on the left side of the right foot, touching the ground if possible.
5. Now lift your left arm and twisting your torso more to the right, almost looking backwards, bring your left arm to rest on the right leg and move both hands in front of your chest in the prayer pose.
6. Without losing the resting of the left forearm on the right thigh, twist more to bring the right elbow are far as possible towards the ceiling.

Breathing:

1. Normal during hold.

Gaze: Front upwards/infinity

Transition pose: None

Next pose: Warrior I left leg front and bent

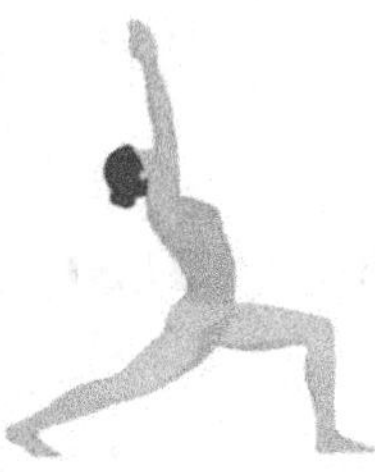

#19

Previous pose: Reverse Warrior

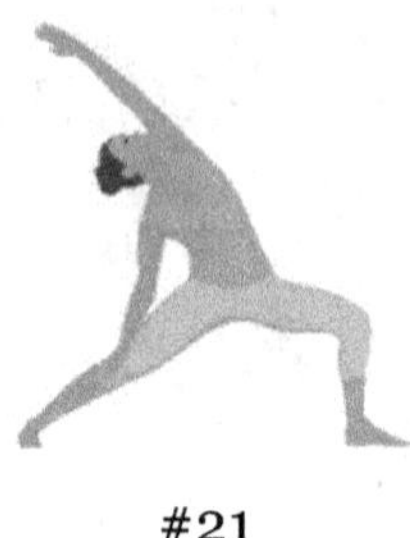

#21

Utthita Parsvakonasana

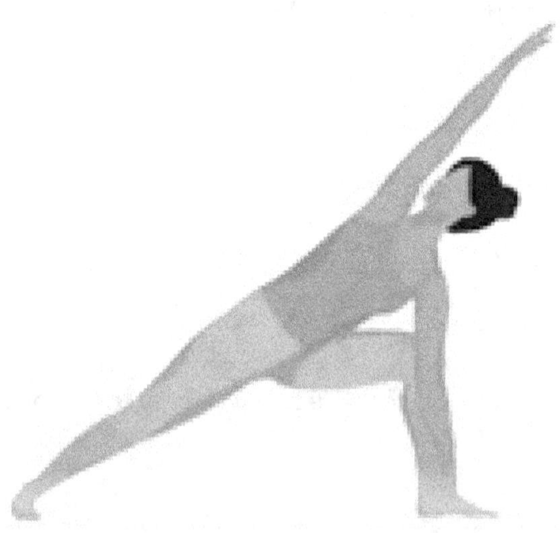

EXTENDED SIDE ANGLE POSE (left leg bent)
#21a

21a. EXTENDED SIDE ANGLE POSE (left leg bent)

1.   From the mountain pose, spread your legs shoulder or more apart.
2.   Turn your left leg and foot outward 90 degrees so your toes point to the left side.
3.   Bend your left knee until your left thigh is parallel to the floor. Keep your left knee directly over your left heel.
4.   Bending to the left from the waist, bring your left arm in front of the left leg and lower it as far as you can, preferably with the left palm on the floor just in front of the left foot.
5.   Now raise and straighten your right arm in the direction of the left toes with your arm touching the right ear.
6.   Look upwards while holding this pose.

Breathing:

    1. Exhalation on way down.
    2. Normal during hold.

Gaze: Front upwards/infinity

Next pose: Revolved side angle pose left leg bent

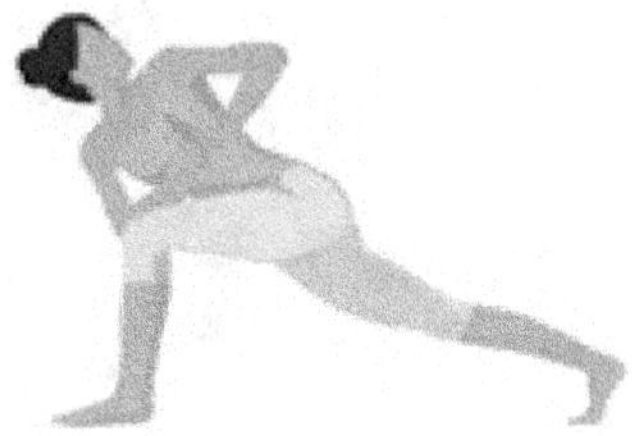

#21b

Previous Pose

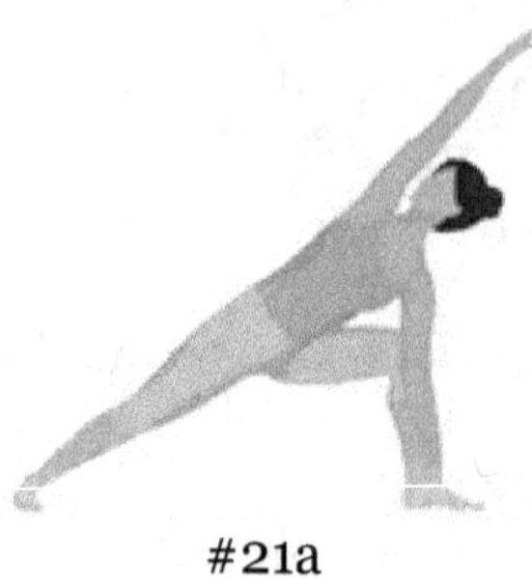

#21a

Parivrtta Parsvakonasana

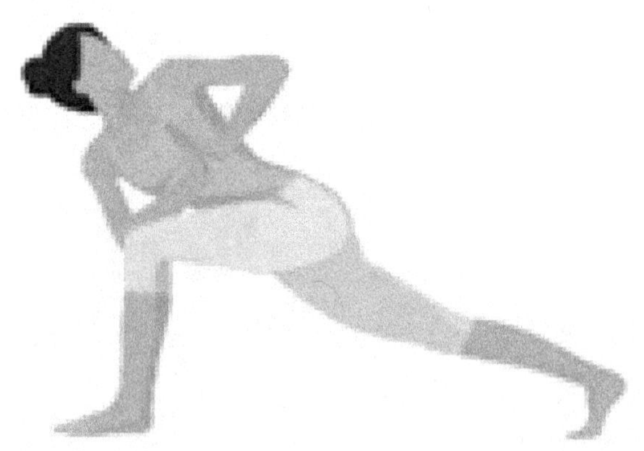

REVOLVED SIDE ANGLE POSE (Left leg bent)
#21b

21b. REVOLVED SIDE ANGLE POSE (Left leg bent)

1. From the mountain pose, spread your legs shoulder or more apart.
2. Turn your left leg and foot outward 90 degrees so your toes point to the left side.
3. Bend your left knee until your left thigh is parallel to the floor. Keep your left knee directly over your left heel.
4. Bending your torso leftwards and downwards, bring your right arm in on the right side of the left foot, touching the ground if possible.
5. Now lift your right arm and twisting your torso more to the left, almost looking backwards, bring your right arm to rest on the left leg and move both hands in front of your chest in the prayer pose.
6. Without losing the resting of the right forearm on the left thigh, twist more to bring the left elbow are far as possible towards the ceiling.

Breathing:

1. Normal during hold.

Gaze: Front upwards/infinity or hands

Next Pose: Warrior II Right leg forward

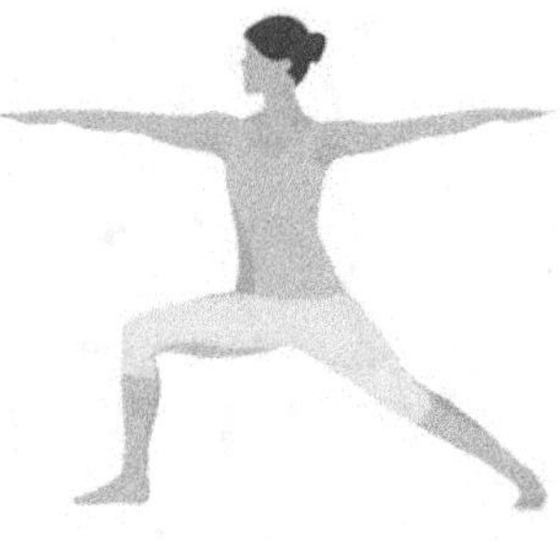

#22

Previous Pose

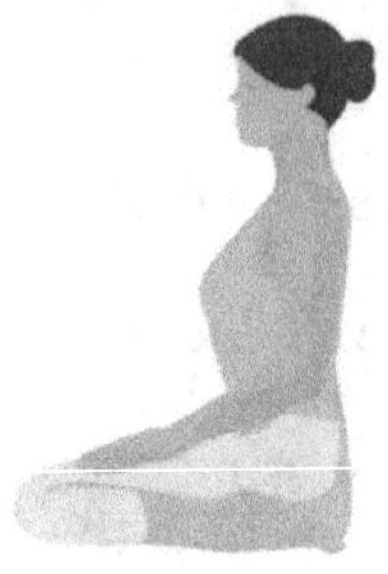

#26

Vakrasana

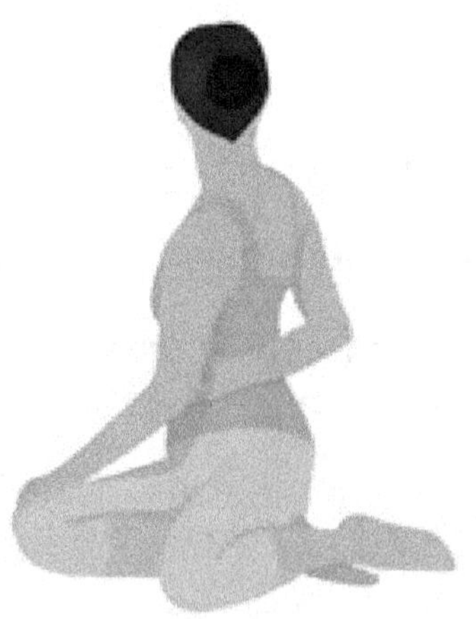

HALF SPINAL TWIST POSE (Right side twist)
#26a

26a.HALF SPINAL TWIST POSE (Right side twist)

1. Start from the *Vajrasana* pose. Your palms are face down on the knees in front of you.
2. Move the left leg and knee leftwards and backwards while the left foot stays in touch with the right foot, behind the body.
3. Twisting the torso rightwards and backwards, move the right hand behind the chest and the left hand on top of the right knee.
4. Twist rightwards and backwards more so that the right hand can hold the left elbow, if possible, behind the back.
5. Hold this pose.

Breathing:

1.Normal during hold.

Gaze: right/infinity

Next pose: Half spinal twist left side

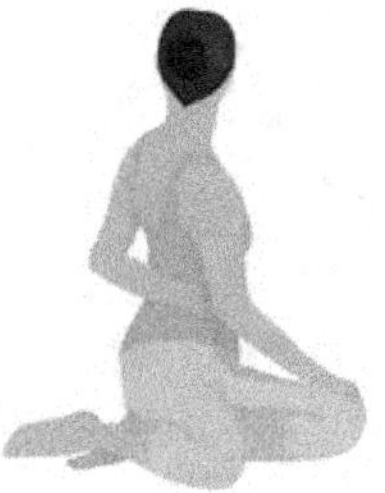

#26b

Previous Pose

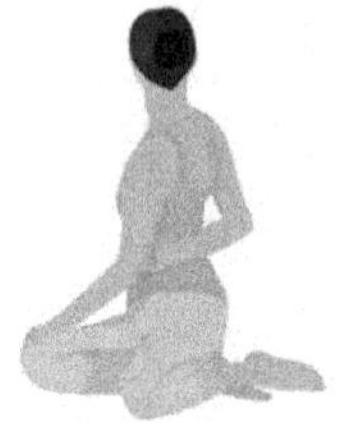

#26a

Vakrasana

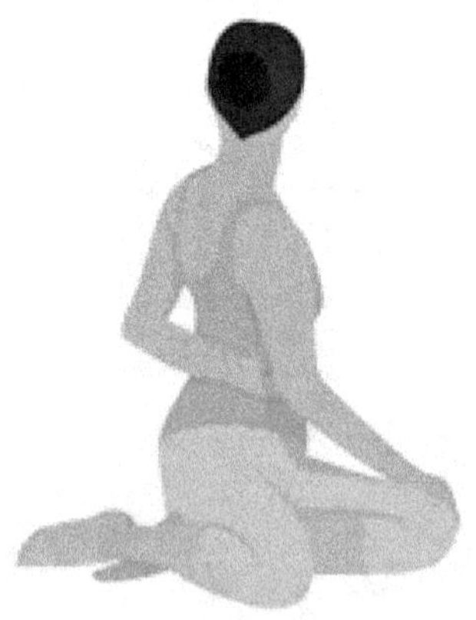

HALF SPINAL TWIST POSE (Left side twist)
#26b

26b. HALF SPINAL TWIST POSE (Left side twist)

1.   Start from the Vajrasana pose. Your palms are face down on the knees in front of you.
2.   Move the right leg and knee rightwards and backwards while the right foot stays in touch with the left foot, behind the body.
3.   Twisting the torso leftwards and backwards, move the left hand behind the chest and the right hand on top of the left knee.
4.   Twist leftwards and backwards more so that the left hand can hold the right elbow, if possible, behind the back.
5.   Hold this pose.

Breathing:

1.   Normal during hold.

Gaze: left/infinity

Next pose: Easy Pose

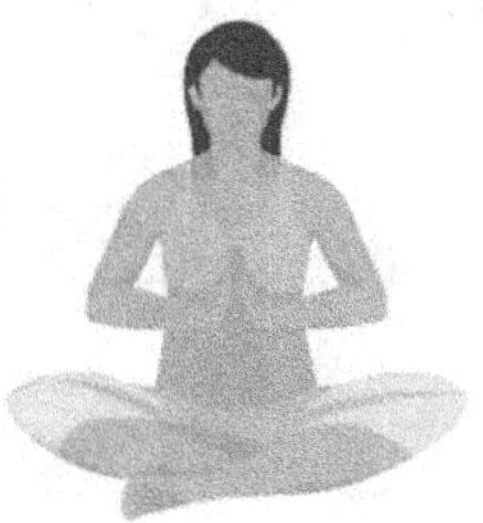

#27

Previous Pose

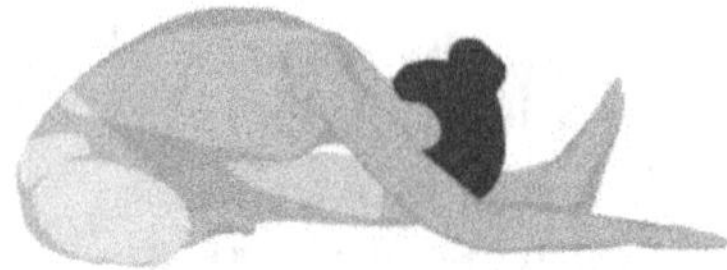

#31

Parivrtta Janu Sirsasana

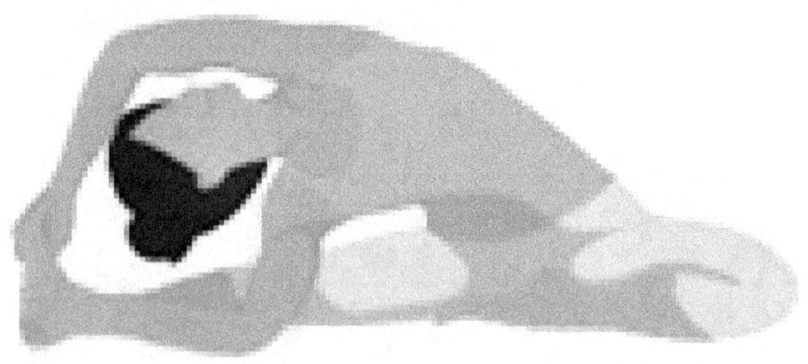

REVOLVED HEAD TO KNEE POSE (Right side)
#31a

31a. REVOLVED HEAD TO KNEE POSE (Right side)

1. Start with the *dandasana* pose.
2. Holding the left knee with the left arm, bend the left knee and holding the left foot with the right hand, pull the foot against the inside of the right leg.
3. The legs stay touching the floor and the right leg is kept straight.
4. Now exhaling, twist your torso to the left and bend your waist towards the right.
5. Stretch your right arm on the inside of the right leg and try to catch the right foot.
6. The left arm goes over the head and similarly tries to catch the right foot.
7. Face upwards and hold this pose.

Breathing:

1. Exhalation on twist and ben.
2. Inhalation on stretch.
3. Normal during hold.

Gaze: upwards/infinity.

Next pose: Revolved head to knee left side

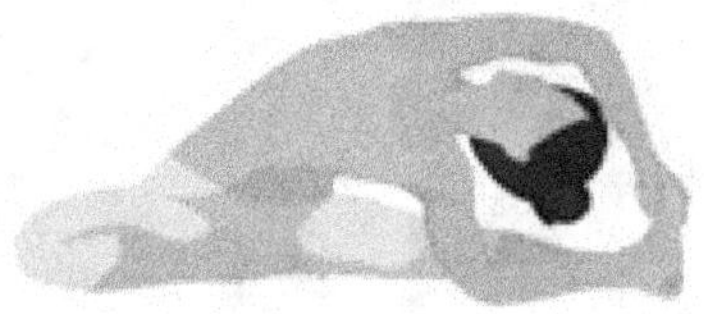

#31b

Previous Pose

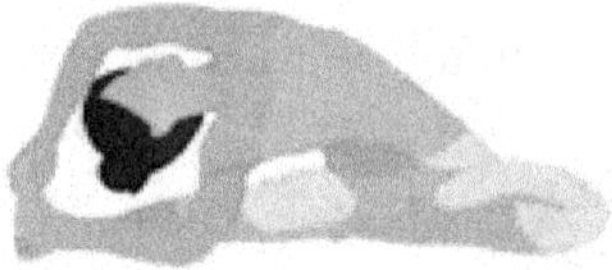

#31a

Parivrtta Janu Sirsasana

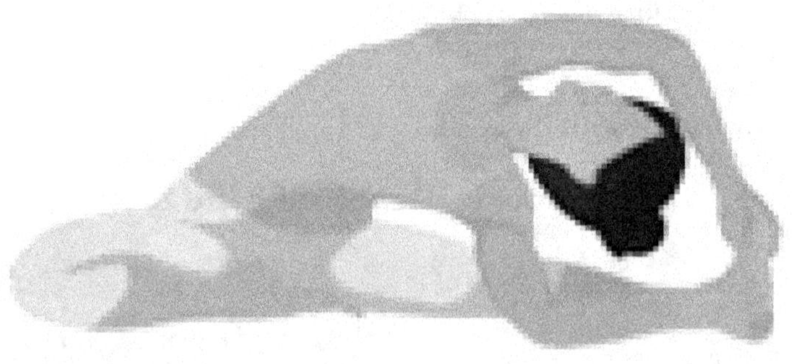

REVOLVED HEAD TO KNEE POSE (Left side)
#31b

31b. REVOLVED HEAD TO KNEE POSE (Left side)

1. Start with the *dandasana* pose.
2. Holding the right knee with the right arm, bend the right knee and holding the right foot with the left hand, pull the foot against the inside of the left leg.
3. The legs stay touching the floor and the left leg is kept straight.
4. Now exhaling, twist your torso to the right and bend your waist towards the left.
5. Stretch your left arm on the inside of the left leg and try to catch the left foot.
6. The right arm goes over the head and similarly tries to catch the left foot.
7. Face upwards and hold this pose.

Breathing:

1. Exhalation on twist and ben.
2. Inhalation on stretch.
3. Normal during hold.

Gaze: upwards/infinity.

Next pose: Thunderbolt Pose

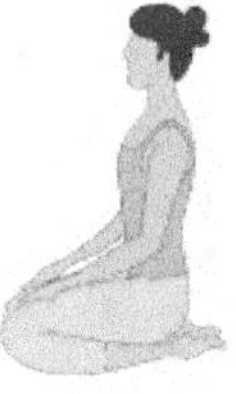

#32

Previous Pose

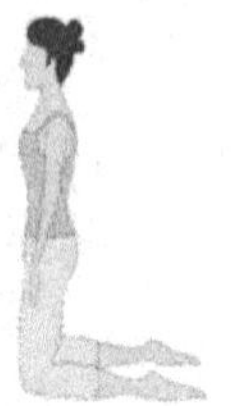

#36

Ustrasana

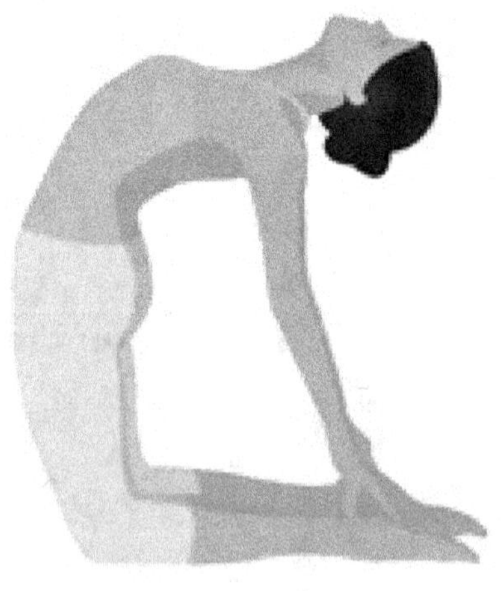

CAMEL POSE
#36a

36a. CAMEL POSE

1. Start in the standing thunderbolt pose.
2. Leaning back, place your hands on the back of your buttocks, with the fingers pointing to the floor.
3. If you can go further, slowly slide your hands further down and see if you can touch the heels with each hand.
4. The chest should be open, and the gaze should be to the ceiling.
5. Hold this pose.

Breathing:

1. Inhalation during the back bend.
2. Normal during hold.

Gaze: upwards/infinity

Next pose: Gate Latch right leg

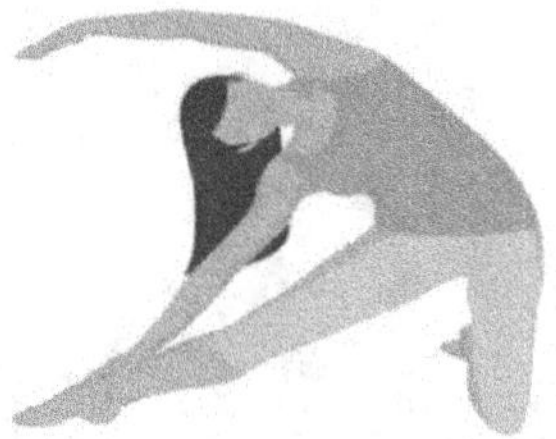

#37

Previous Pose

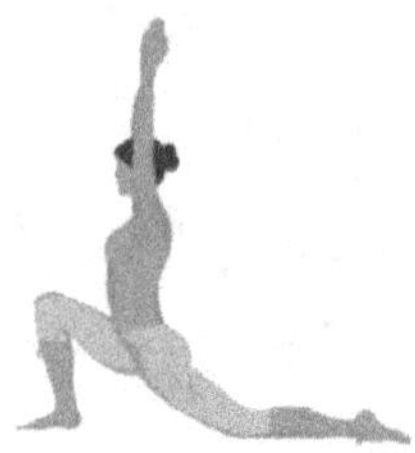

#40

Modified Anjaneyasana

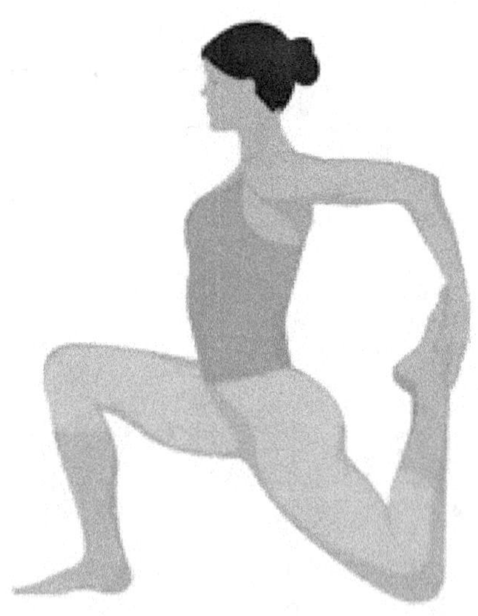

MODIFIED LOW LUNGE (Right knee front and bent)
#40a

40a. MODIFIED LOW LUNGE (Right knee front and bent)

1. Start from the low lunge pose with the right knee bent and forward.
2. Bring both arms down by the side.
3. Bend the left leg at the knee and bring the foot up and towards the left buttock.
4. Use your left hand to lay the palmer surface on the upper surface of the left foot.
5. The right arm stays on the right-side flush with the body, with the palms against the right side of the body.
6. Hold this pose.
7. To come out of pose, straighten your left leg again.
8. Slowly bend forwards and bring your hands down and put your palms on the floor besides the right knee. P
9. Pushing your palms downwards, slowly stretch your right leg backwards and slowly raising your torso, come into the downward facing dog pose.

Breathing:

1. Normal during hold.

Gaze: Front/infinity

Next Pose: Low lunge with left knee bent

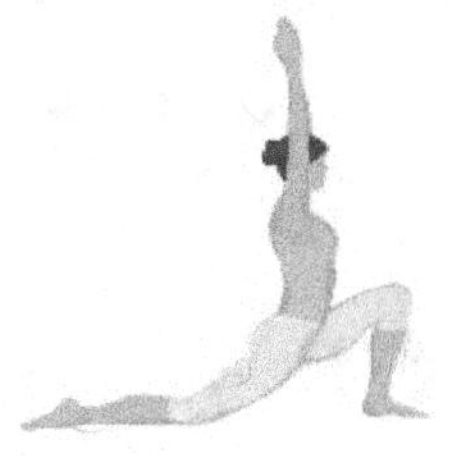

#41

Previous Pose

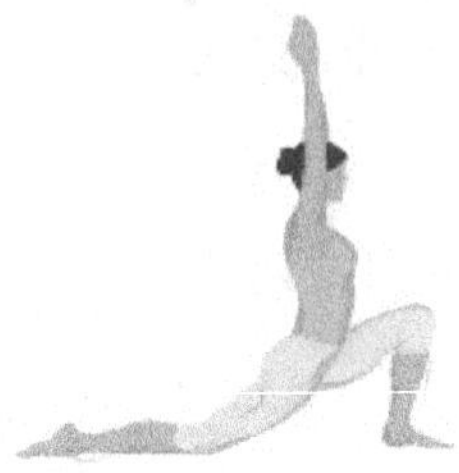

#41

Modified Anjaneyasana

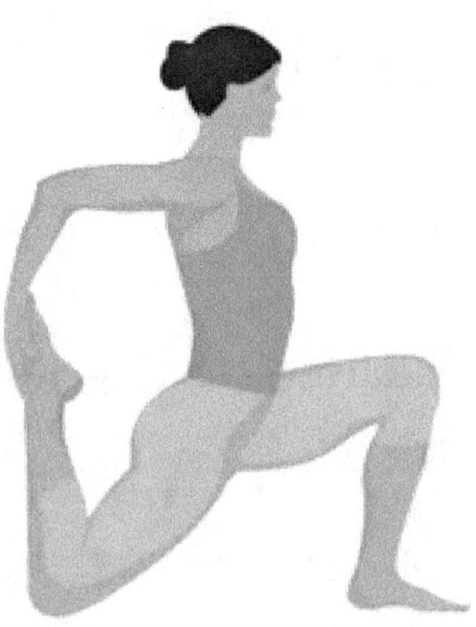

MODIFIED LOW LUNGE (left knee front and bent)
#41a

41a. MODIFIED LOW LUNGE (left knee front and bent)

1.   Start from the low lunge pose with the right knee bent and forward.
2.   Bring both arms down by the side.
3.   Bend the left leg at the knee and bring the foot up and towers the left buttock.
4.   Use your left hand to lay the palmer surface on the upper surface of the left foot.
5.   The right arm stays on the right-side flush with the body, with the palms against the right side of the body.
6.   Hold this pose.
7.   To come out of pose, straighten your left leg again.
8.   Slowly bend forwards and bring your hands down and put your palms on the floor besides the right knee. P
9.   Pushing your palms downwards, slowly stretch your right leg backwards and slowly raising your torso, come into the downward facing dog pose.

Breathing:

1.   Normal during hold.

Gaze: Front/infinity or hands

Transition pose: None

Next Pose: Reverse Corpse Pose

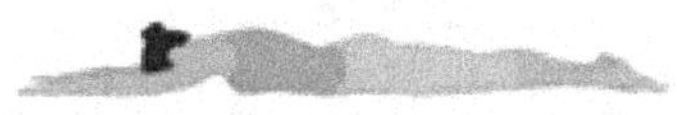

#41b

Previous Pose

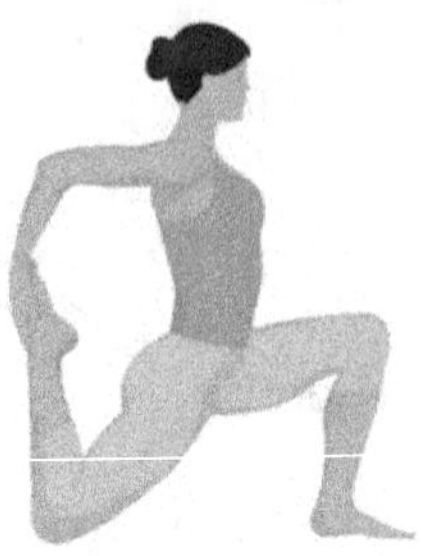

#41a

Advasana

REVERSE CORPSE POSE
#41b

41b. REVERSE CORPSE POSE

1. Bringing your arms forward and downwards, slowly lower your torso and move your legs backwards.
2. Lie down on the belly.
3. Place the fore head on the ground.
4. Move both arms forward over the head.
5. The palms of the hands rest on the floor.
6. The legs should also be stretched back.
7. Relax and breathe normally.

Breathing: Normal during pose

Gaze: floor

Next Pose: Sphynx Pose

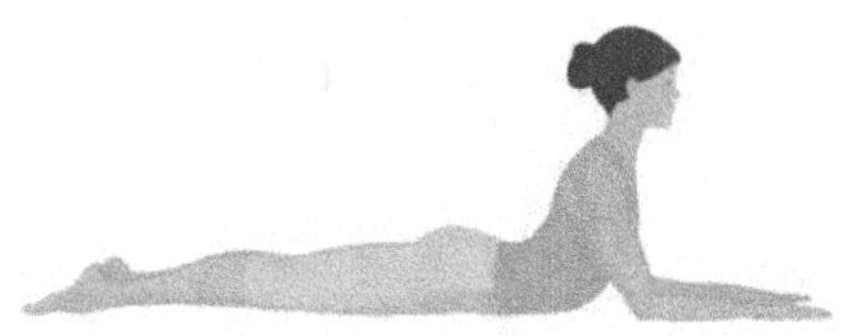

#42

Previous Pose

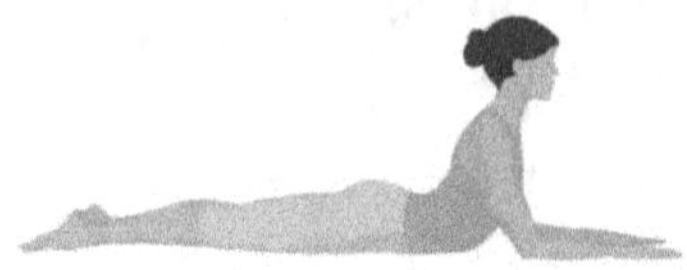

#42

Ardha Pincha Mayurasana

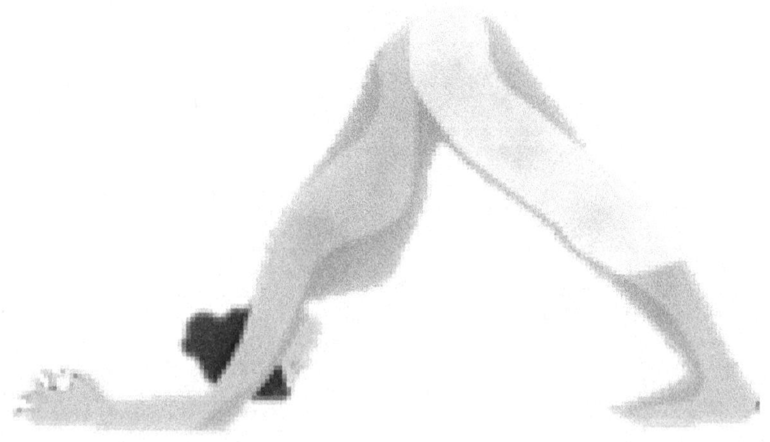

DOLPHIN POSE
#42a

42a. DOLPHIN POSE

1. Start in the sphynx pose.
2. Your forearms are on the floor and your elbows and shoulders are in a parallel line.
3. Now raise your back upwards and straighten your back legs. The feet are flat on the ground and facing forwards.
4. Now raise your shoulders away from ears, but keep your elbows and forearms on the floor.
5. After that walk your feet in towards your arms.

Breathing

1. Normal during hold

Gaze: Back legs

Next Pose: Dolphin Plank

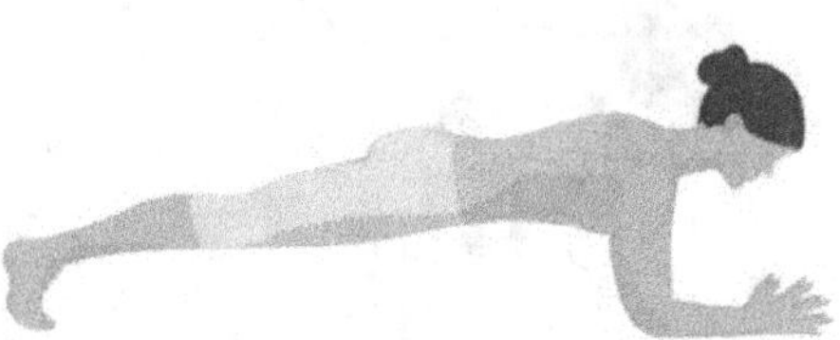

#43

Previous Pose

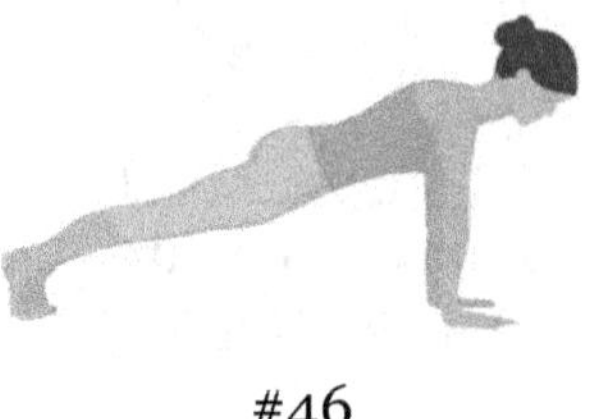

#46

Chaturanga Dandasana

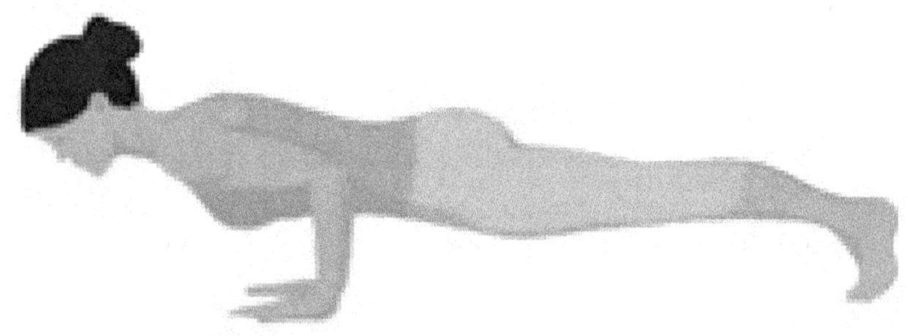

FOUR LIMBED STAFF POSE
#46a

46a. FOUR LIMBED STAFF POSE

1. You are in the downward plank pose – starting pose.
2. The hands should be under your shoulders and feet hip-distance apart.
3. While exhaling lower your body toward the floor.
4. Keep your elbows tucked in toward your sides and keep your legs straight. You remain on your toes.
5. You are at right angles at the elbow and the wrist.
6. The forearm is perpendicular to the ground while the upper arm and the body is parallel to the ground.
7. You are looking at the floor in front of you.

Breathing

1. Exhalation during lowering the torso.
2. Normal breathing during the hold.

Gaze: Floor

Next Pose: Cat Pose

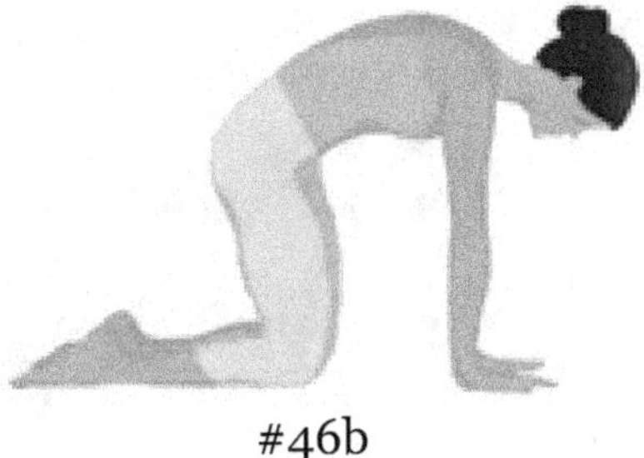

#46b

Previous Pose

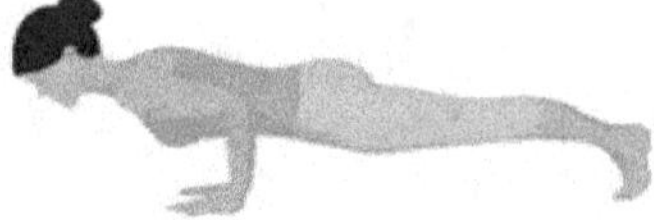

#46a

Marjaiasana

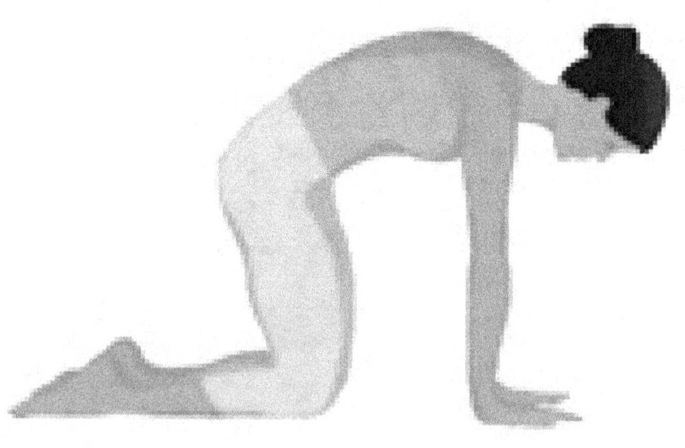

CAT POSE
#46b

46b. CAT POSE

1. From the four-limbed staff pose, slowly lower you lower legs on the floor.
2. The thighs stay upright with the hips directly above your bent knees.
3. Straighten your arms so that they are perpendicular to the floor and the shoulders are directly above the bent wrists.
4. Exhaling, draw your belly to your spine and round your back toward the ceiling.
5. You are now looking like a cat stretching its back.
6. You can let the head drop forward gently.
7. Hold the pose.

Breathing:

1. Exhalation during the back bend.
2. Normal during hold.

Gaze: floor/hands

Next Pose: Cow Pose

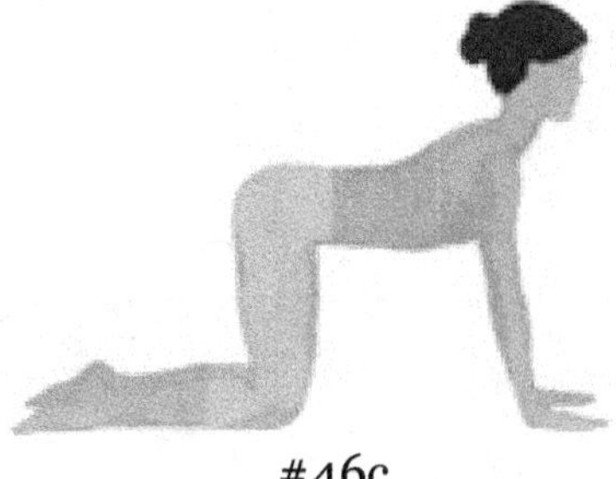

#46c

Previous Pose

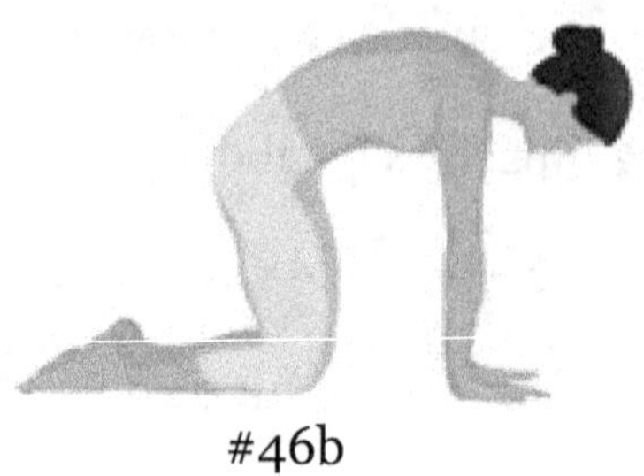

#46b

Bitilasana

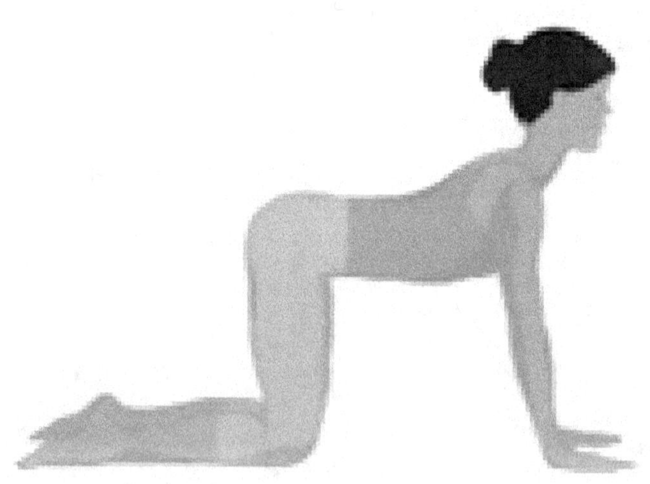

COW POSE
#46c

46c. COW POSE

1. From the four-limbed staff pose, slowly lower you lower legs on the floor.
2. The thighs stay upright with the hips directly above your bent knees.
3. Straighten your arms so that they are perpendicular to the floor and the shoulders are directly above the bent wrists.
4. You are now in the cat pose.
5. Inhaling, drop your belly towards the floor so that your back is concave upwards.
6. The head moves upwards and you are now seeing up and front.
7. Hold the pose.

Breathing:

1. Inhalation during belly drop.
2. Normal during the hold.

Gaze: upwards/front

Next Pose: Locust

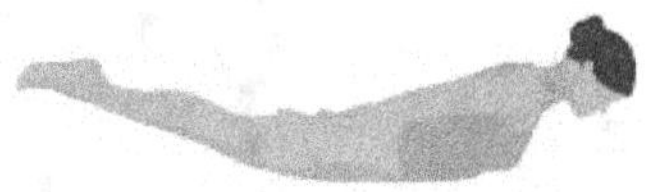

#47

Previous Pose

#49

Modified Anantasana

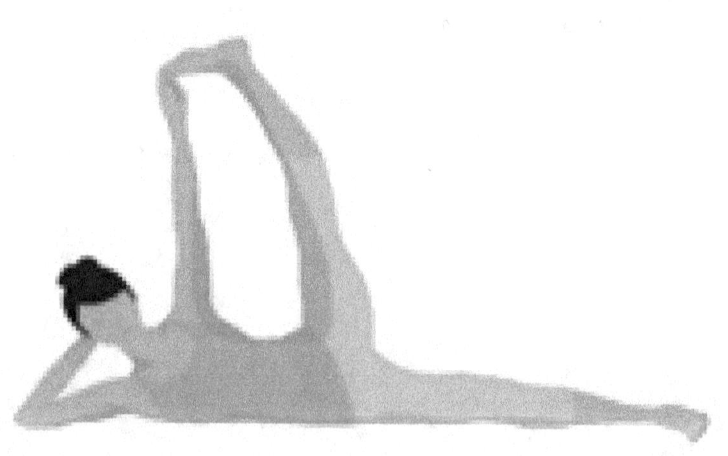

RECLINING BUDDHA (Right side with Left leg up)
#49a

49a. RECLINING BUDDHA (Right side with Left leg up)

1. You are in the reclining Buddha facing with your right arm under your head and your left arm on your left hip.
2. Slowly raise your left leg upwards and grab the left toes with your left hand.
3. Gradually raise the arm and leg as far up as possible.
4. During this entire exercise, the left arm and left leg remain in the same 'line' as the rest of the body.
5. Hold this pose. Breathe normally.

Breathing: Normal during hold

Gaze: front (right/facing side)/infinity

Next Pose: Side Plank Right Side

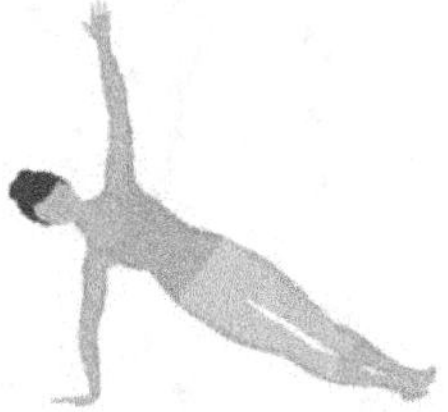

#50

Previous Pose

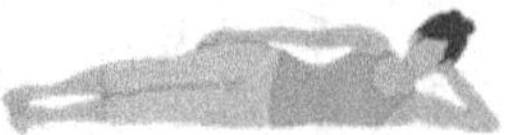

#51

Modified Anantasana

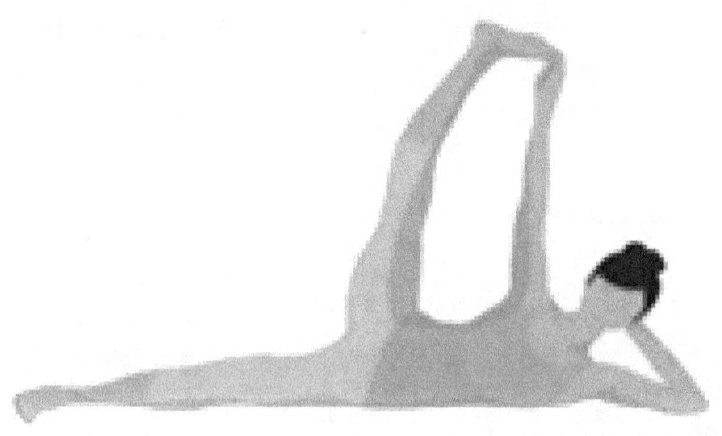

RECLINING BUDDHA (Left side with Right leg up)
#51a

51a. RECLINING BUDDHA (Left side with Right leg up)

1.   You are in the reclining Buddha facing with your left arm under your head and your right arm on your right hip.
2.   Slowly raise your right leg upwards and grab the right toes with your right hand.
3.   Gradually raise the arm and leg as far up as possible.
4.   During this entire exercise, the right arm and right leg remain in the same 'line' as the rest of the body.
5.   Hold this pose. Breathe normally.

Breathing: Normal during hold

Gaze: front (right/facing side) infinity

Next Pose: Side Plank Left Side

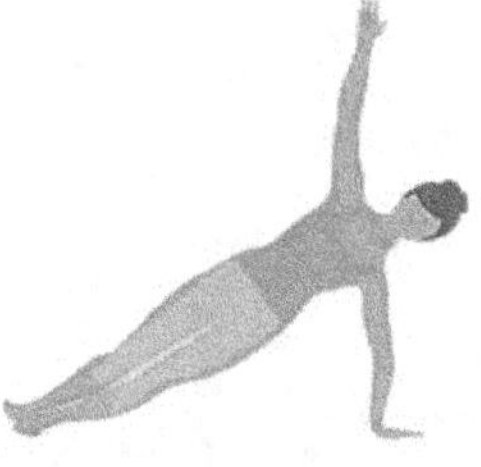

#52

Previous Pose

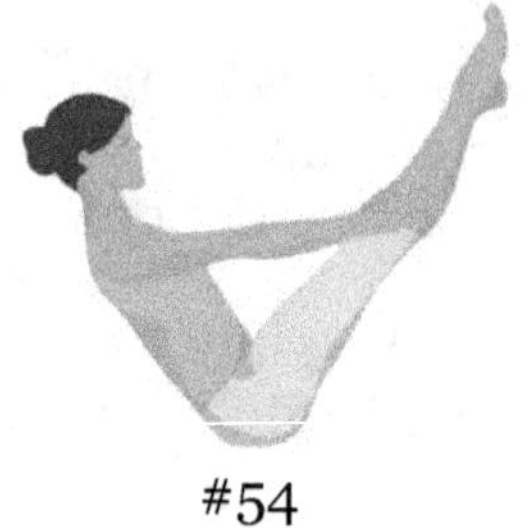

#54

Matsyasana

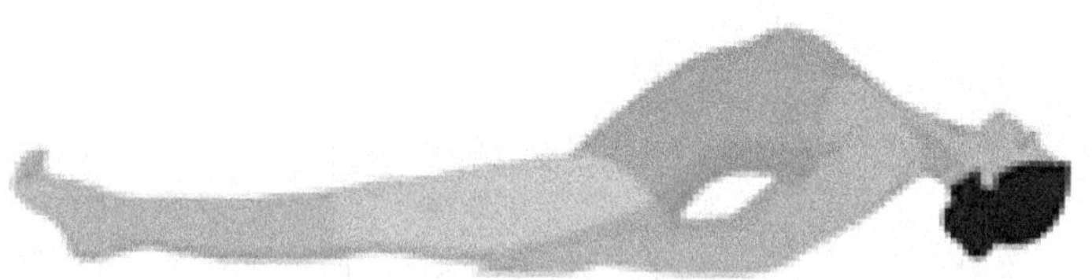

FISH POSE
#54a

54a. FISH POSE

1. Begin in the corpse pose with your arms resting alongside your body, palms down.
2. Press your forearms and elbows into the floor and lift your chest to create an arch in your upper back.
3. Lifting your shoulder blades, raise the upper torso off the floor.
4. Now tilt your head back and bring the crown of your head to the floor. The head should be bearing very little weight.
5. The legs stay in the same position as when started.
6. Hold this pose.

Breathing:

1. Inhalation during lifting the torso.
2. Normal during pose

Gaze: upwards/infinity

Next Pose: Happy Baby Pose

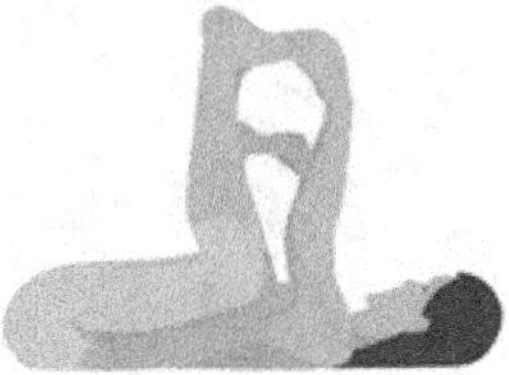

#55

Previous Pose

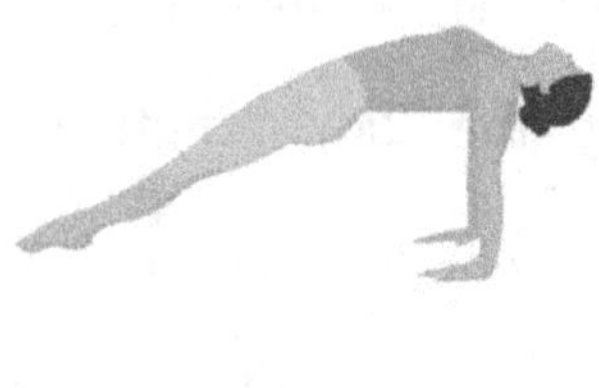

#58

Supta Baddha Konasana

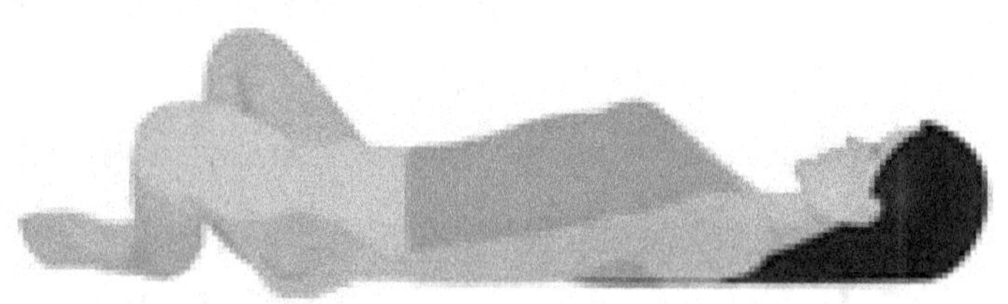

RECLINING BOUND ANGLE POSE
#58a

58a. RECLINING BOUND ANGLE POSE

1. Start in the corpse pose.
2. Move your arms about 30 degrees outwards and let them relax with the palms facing up.
3. Bend your knees and draw your heels in toward your pelvis/groin. Press the soles of your feet together and let your knees drop open to both sides.
4. Hold this pose.

Breathing:

1. Normal during hold.

Gaze: upwards/infinity

Next Pose: Supine Spinal Twist Right

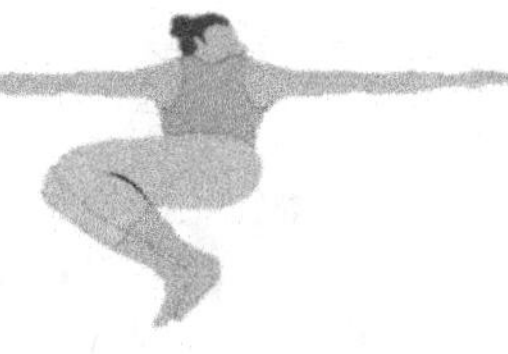

#59

Previous Pose

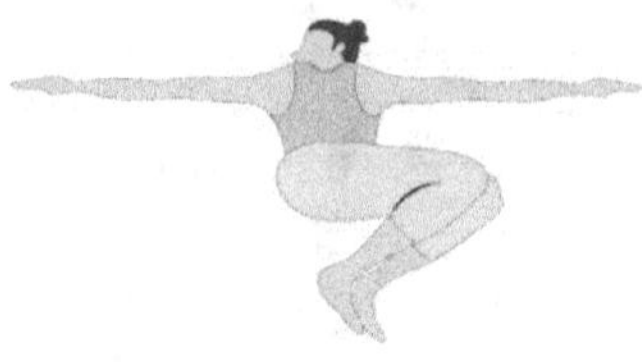

#60

Salamba Sarvangasana

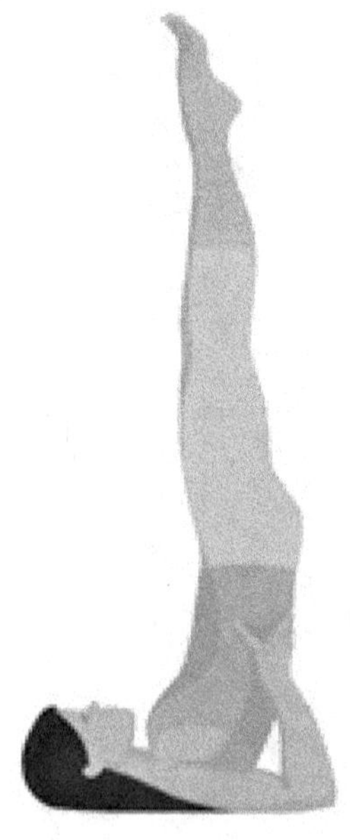

SHOULDER STAND (Supported)
#60a

60a. SHOULDER STAND (Supported)

1. Begin in the corpse pose.
2. You are lying flat on your back with your legs extended straight and your arms at your sides, palms down.
3. Now bend your knees and place the soles of your feet flat on the floor.
4. Bend your elbows and place your hands on your lower back with your fingertips pointing up toward the feet.
5. Inhaling, lift your legs and torso upwards, (with the help of the hands on the lower back) initially the knees towards the face and then straightening them so that the torso and legs are perpendicular to the ground.
6. The head and upper spine should be in one line.
7. Look at your feet.
8. Hold the pose.

Breathing:

1. Inhalation during the body lift.
2. Normal during hold.

Gaze: upwards/feet

Next Pose: Corpse Pose

b. **TOTAL BODY RELAXATION**

Follow this by Total Body Relaxation mentioned in Sequence I.

c. **PRANAYAMA** (Sequence II - additions)

Add these two breathing exercises to the previous ones mentioned with the 60-pose sequence I: Your total breathing exercise time increases to 15 minutes:

1. Ujjai Breath (exercise) 2 minutes
2. Chakra breathing (exercise) 3 minutes

1. **Ujjayi Breath**

Ujjayi breathing warms your body. It can help release emotions and calm your mind. It should be done seated. Breathe nice and easy through your nose. Now take an inhalation through your nose that is deeper than normal – fill your lungs completely. Exhale slowly through your nose while constricting the muscles in the back of your throat. This should create a sound audible to you (like a coarse aaaahh), but not audible a few feet away. Each inhalation and exhalation should take about 10 seconds. Do this exercise for 6 times or more.

2. **Chakra breathing**

Chakras are seven in number and have been described before. They represent wheels spinning in response to energy at various key locations in the body. Yogis have assigned them with different colors and properties. To recapitulate, these are:

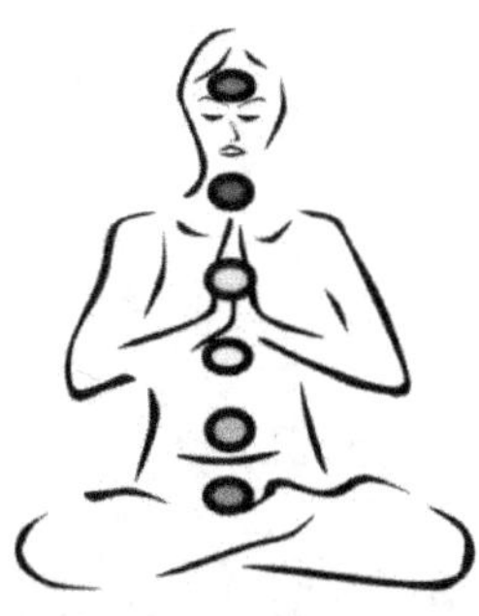

The Root Chakra (red) – base of spine
The Sacral Chakra (orange) – just below navel
The Solar Plexus Chakra (yellow) – above the navel
The Heart Chakra (green) – located at heart level
The Throat Chakra (blue) - at throat level
The 3rd Eye Chakra (indigo) – just above eyebrows
The Crown Chakra (violet) – top of the head

Chakra breathing is ideally done standing up in the *Tadasana* pose. The idea is to open up these chakras and allow the wheels from changing from sluggish or overactive spinning to a balanced spinning – which allows energy to travel and radiate calmly and properly.

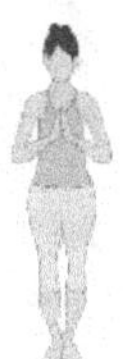

Breathe normally through the nose. Then while inhaling, direct the breath to the first chakra – root chakra. Exhaling, let the breath leave the same chakra. This should take about 10 seconds for both inhalation and exhalation. Next breath move up to the second chakra – the sacral chakra and so on. Once you reach the crown chakra – reverse the process and start coming down till you reach the root chakra – and then start the process again going up and so on...

d. **DHAYANA** (Sequence II – additions)

"To a mind that is still, the whole universe surrenders."

Lao-Tzu

Add these two meditations to the ones in Sequence I. Your meditation time increases by another 15 minutes to a total of 20 minutes:

1. Chakra meditation (5 minutes)

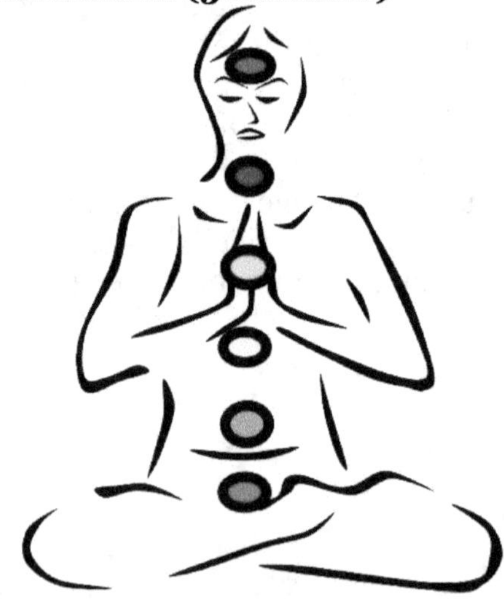

Again, there are seven energy centers (Chakras) in our body:

The Root Chakra (red) – base of spine

The Sacral Chakra (orange) – just below navel

The Solar Plexus Chakra (yellow) – above the navel

The Heart Chakra (green) – located at heart level

The Throat Chakra (blue) - at throat level

The 3rd Eye Chakra (indigo) – just above eyebrows

The Crown Chakra (violet) – top of the head

With quiet breathing in and out through the nostril, imagine the energy in the breath going to the root chakra and making the red wheel glow. The energy flows in with each inhalation and then the breath leaves the chakra with each exhalation. Do this with each chakra in turn, from the root to the third eye. The crown chakra is not involved in this exercise. Each chakra should take approximately 10 seconds. Do five cycles for a total of five minutes.

6. Mindfulness Meditation (10 minutes)

Sit comfortably with legs crossed and the palms facing down on the thighs. Clear your mind and start listening and feeling your breath. The breathing is normal. While doing this, you will be distracted by thoughts – just observe them without making any judgements and let them pass. If you appear to get involved with some thought – just return to the breath observation. It is natural for the mind to wander again – but you know what to do. Do not force 'thoughtlessness', but allow the thoughts to come and go. Just remember to get back into your meditation if distracted. You can do the same thing by observing the body. Do this for ten minutes.

The meditation period should follow the breathing session. If you fall off into sleep - fine. Meditation can also be done independently - before any preceding asanas or breathing exercises. Make sure the place, pose and conditions are kept as close to as possible to those listed under yoga and pranayama.

"Renew thyself completely each day; do it again, and again, and forever."

Cherokee Saying

9. ADVERSE EFFECTS OF YOGA

'Primum non nocere' – 'first, to do no harm'

Auguste François Chomel (1788–1858)

Complementary or alternate medicine (CAM) is popular I the US. One government survey indicated that approximately 38% of U.S. adults aged 18 years and over and approximately 12% of children use some form of CAM[1]. Yoga was one of the top 10 complementary and integrative health approaches used among U.S. adults according to the 2007 National Health Interview Survey[2]. It is extremely popular in general population for its divers physical and mental benefits in healthy people[3]. It is also increasingly being used in diseases as an adjunct therapeutic modality[4].

Swain and McGwin looked at data from the National Electronic Injury Surveillance System from 2001 to 2014 for yoga related injuries. Researchers found that of the 29,590 yoga-related injuries seen in hospital emergency departments during this period, the most frequent area injured was the trunk (46.6%) and sprain/strain (45.0%). The injury rate was higher in those aged 65 years or more (57.9/100,000) compared with those aged 18 to 44 years (11.9/100,000) and 45 to 64 years (17.7/100,000) in 2014[5]. Fishman and group surveyed more than 1300 yoga teachers worldwide. They found that yoga injuries usually involved the neck, lower back, knee, shoulder, and wrist. According to them, the most common causes were poor technique, poor instruction, previous injury, and excess effort[6]. They reported that particular injuries were linked with particular asanas. According to them, neck injuries were commonly attributed to *sarvangasana* (shoulder stand) while lower-back injuries were associated with forward bends, twists, and backbends. Shoulder and wrist injuries were usually due to *adho mukha svanasana* (downward-facing dog) and different plank poses (e.g., *chaturanga dandasana -*

four-limbed staff pose and *vasisthasana* - side plank pose). The knees were more likely to be injured in *virabhadrasana* (warrior pose I and II), and *virasana* (hero's pose) .

While most injuries are minor[7], serious injuries such as bone fractures[8] and tendon/ligament injuries[9] may occur. Non-musculoskeletal injuries have also been reported[10,11]. According to one study, injuries lead to stoppage in less than 1% of yoga participants[12].

In general, adverse effects with yoga practice are uncommon. The National Institute of Health in the US recommends that yoga should however be practiced with a well-educated instructor. Elderly people and those with limitations need to practice extra caution with yoga practice. I would therefore also recommend that you fine tune your poses with a certified yoga instructor – to avoid injuries.

10. PARTING THOUGHTS

"Do not feel lonely. The entire universe is inside of you."

Rumi

Yoga Sutras describe 8 limbs of yoga – including asanas, pranayama and dhyana.

Yoga posture (asana) practice will bring you strength, flexibility and improved coordination. Breathing exercises (pranayama) will bring clean fresh energy (prana) into your body and get rid of the toxic energy (apana). Meditation (dhyana) will help remove or restrain unnecessary and often damaging brain activity constantly running in the background. It will calm your mind and help you relax on the inside. I will recommend that you visit a yoga class so that a certified yoga teacher can help fine tune your poses, for better physiological benefit.

B.K.S. Iyengar in his book, 'Light on Life' said that when faced with different personalities and their often pathological emotions, one should cultivate the following approaches:

1. Maitri: friendship towards those who are happy.

2. Karuna: compassion towards those who are in sorrow.

3. Mudita: joy towards those who are victorious.

4. Upeksa: indifference or neutrality towards those who are full of vices.

The latter emotional approach may often be the best way of handling the toxic milieu of emotionally disturbed vibes you may face in life.

Yoga is an ancient practice that has been able to survive through the years. While most of us practice just one part of yoga, we often don't realize that there are in fact 8 limbs to the practice of yoga. The Sage Patanjali wrote the Yoga Sutras (sutras = observations about general truth), and this compilation in Sanskrit contains 196 sutras. While the exact date of the sutras creation is hotly contested amongst yoga scholars, the text itself is incredibly old. The text lays out an 8-limb path of yoga, with details of how to practice, ways to treat oneself, ways to treat others and guidance to remain on the path of spirituality.

These eight limbs were mentioned earlier. To repeat, these are:

- Yama – Morality

- Niyama – Personal Observances

- Asana – Body Movement

- Pranayama – Control of Prana through Breathing

- Pratyahara – Sense Control

- Dharana – Concentration

- Dhyana – Meditation

- Samadhi – Union with the Almighty

By being aware and mindful, you can direct your life into transforming you into a better person. With regular practice of the three limbs of yoga descried in this book, and with acceptance of yamas and niyamas and practice of prtyahara and dharna, one can attain samadhi - or eternal internal bliss. Do not expect immediate changes – but with time you will change yourself into someone you will like – and be proud of.

Make your journey through this phase of life less stressful and less negative - and glide through it with a new broader understanding of the purpose of life. An understanding that you are going through this physical life only once, an understanding that both good things and bad things are inevitable in everyone's life, an understanding that you want to stay happy during this journey despite the peaks and nadirs, an understanding that you are connected with the universal energy through the spirit, and an understanding that you can achieve most things you desire through energy received through this connection from the universal source. All you need to do is align and vibrate with the cosmic energy.

"To a mind that is still, the whole universe surrenders."

Lao-Tzu

11. REFERENCES

HEALTH WOES OF AMERICA

1. https://ourworldindata.org/life-expectancy/ - (accessed 10/14/17)
2. https://www.elderweb.com/book/appendix/1900-2000-changes-life-expectancy-united-states/ - (accessed 10/14/17).
3. https://www.washingtonpost.com/national/health-science/us-life-expectancy-declines-for-the-first-time-since-1993/2016/12/07/7dcdc7b4-bc93-11e6-91ee-1adddfe36cbe_story.html?utm_term=.540fe7097477 – (accessed 10/14/17).
4. https://www.theatlantic.com/health/archive/2016/03/less-than-3-percent-of-americans-live-a-healthy-lifestyle/475065/ - (accessed 10/14/17) .
5. https://www.theatlantic.com/health/archive/2016/03/less-than-3-percent-of-americans-live-a-healthy-lifestyle/475065/ - (accessed 10/14/17).
6. https://www.cdc.gov/nchs/fastats/leading-causes-of-death.htm - (accessed 10/14/17).
7. https://newsroom.heart.org/news/new-statistics-show-one-of-every-three-u-s-deaths-caused-by-cardiovascular-disease.
8. https://www.cancer.org/research/cancer-facts-statistics/all-cancer-facts-figures/cancer-facts-figures-2017.html (accessed May 24, 2017).
9. https://www.cancer.org/research/cancer-facts-statistics/all-cancer-facts-figures/cancer-facts-figures-2017.html (accessed May 24, 2017).
10. http://www.nationalbreastcancer.org/breast-cancer-facts.
11. https://www.nimh.nih.gov/health/statistics/prevalence/any-mental-illness-ami-among-us-adults.shtml - (accessed 10/14/17).
12. https://www.nimh.nih.gov/health/statistics/prevalence/any-mental-illness-ami-among-us-adults.shtml - (accessed 10/14/17).
13. http://www.mentalhealthamerica.net/issues/state-mental-health-america -(accessed 10/14/17).
14. https://www.psychologytoday.com/blog/the-mindful-self-express/201702/americans-just-broke-new-record-stress-and-anxiety - (accessed 10/14/17).
15. https://www.nytimes.com/interactive/2017/06/05/upshot/opioid-epidemic-drug-overdose-deaths-are-rising-faster-than-ever.html.
16. http://www.businessinsider.com/homicide-rates-in-major-us-cities-to-break-records-in-2017-2017-7.
17. https://www.fbi.gov/news/pressrel/press-releases/fbi-releases-2015-crime-statistics (accessed 4/2/18).
18. http://worldhappiness.report/
19. https://www.huffingtonpost.com/entry/american-religion-trends_us_570c21cee4b0836057a235ad - (accessed 10/14/17).

MILLENNIAL HEALTH OUTLOOK

1. Fry R. Fact Tank (Internet): Pew Research Center. May 11, 2015. [Accessed Oct 17 2017]. Available from: http://www.pewresearch.org/fact-tank/2015/05/11/millennials-surpass-gen-xers-as-the-largest-generation-in-u-s-laborforce/.

2. Patten E, Fry R. Fact Tank (Internet): Pew Research Center. Mar 19, 2015. [Accessed Oct 17 2017]. Available from: http://www.pewresearch.org/fact-tank/2015/03/19/how-millennials-compare-with-their-grandparents/.

3. Dews F. Brookings Now (Internet): Brookings. Jul 17, 2014. [Accessed Oct 17 2017]. Available from: https://www.brookings.edu/blog/brookings-now/2014/07/17/brookings-data-now-75-percent-of-2025-workforce-willbe-millennials/.

4. Pew Research Center. Millennials, a Portrait of Generation Next: Confident, Connected, Open to Change. February 2010. http://www.pewsocialtrends.org/files/2010/10/millennials-confident-connected-open-to-change.pdf. Accessed August 3, 2017.

5. Pew Research Center. Millennials: A Portrait of Generation Next. Washington, DC: Pew Research Center; 2010.

6. Gallup-Healthways Well-Being Index from http://www.chicagotribune.com/lifestyles/health/ct-young-americans-unhealthy-and-skinny-20160511-story.html.

7. U.S. Department of Health and Human Services Centers for Disease Control and Prevention. (2008). 2007 National youth risk behavior survey overview. Retrieved August 4, 2009, from http://www.cdc.gov/HealthyYouth/yrbs/pdf/yrbs07_us_overview.pdf.

8. https://www.statista.com/statistics/713338/weight-of-millennials-united-states/.

9. Nicky Broyd. Obesity Risk for Millennials - Medscape - Feb 27, 2018.

10. U.S. Department of Health and Human Services Centers for Disease Control and Prevention. (2008). 2007 National youth risk behavior survey overview. Retrieved August 4, 2009, from http://www.cdc.gov/HealthyYouth/yrbs/pdf/yrbs07_us_overview.pdf.

11. https://www.brit.co/heres-why-millennials-are-so-dedicated-to-practicing-mindfulness/.

12. .http://www.thedatereport.com/dating/trends/cheerful-stat-of-the-day-85-percent-of-relationships-end-in-breakups/

13. https://www.psychologytoday.com/blog/the-mindful-self-express/201503/the-top-4-reasons-relationships-fail)

14. https://www.brit.co/heres-why-millennials-are-so-dedicated-to-practicing-mindfulness/.

15. Audelo, Sarah and Frothingham, Sunny. (September 18 2015). "3.6 Million Millennials Gained Health Insurance in 2014." Center for American Progress. Available at

https://www.americanprogress.org/issues/healthcare/news/2015/09/1
8/121577/3-6-million-millennials-gained-health-insurance-in-2014/

16. https://www.nirsonline.org/2018/02/new-research-finds-95-percent-
of-millennials-not-saving-adequately-for-retirement/.

17. https://www.nirsonline.org/2018/02/new-research-finds-95-percent-
of-millennials-not-saving-adequately-for-retirement/.

18. Wotus, Matt. (September 29 2015). "Millennials More Likely Than
Other Generations to Avoid Seeing a Doctor."
http://genprogress.org/voices/2015/09/29/39979/millennials-more-
likely-than-other-generations-to-avoid-seeing-a-doctor/.

19. Wotus, Matt. (September 29 2015). "Millennials More Likely Than
Other Generations to Avoid Seeing a Doctor."
http://genprogress.org/voices/2015/09/29/39979/millennials-more-
likely-than-other-generations-to-avoid-seeing-a-doctor/.

20. https://www.businesswire.com/news/home/20170517005431/en/Digni
ty-Health-Launches-Take2Mins-Mindfulness-Practice-Fostering.

HEALTH BENEFITS OF YOGA

1. Dunn KD. A review of the literature examining the physiolo.gical
processes underlying the therapeutic benefits of Hatha yoga. Adv Mind
Body Med. 2008 Fall;23(3):10-8.

2. Halder K, Chatterjee A, Pal R, Tomer OS, Saha M. Age related
differences of selected Hatha yoga practices on anthropometric
characteristics, muscular strength and flexibility of healthy individuals.
International Journal of Yoga. 2015;8(1):37-46. doi:10.4103/0973-
6131.146057.

3. Lau C, Yu R, Woo J. Effects of a 12-Week Hatha Yoga Intervention on
Cardiorespiratory Endurance, Muscular Strength and Endurance, and
Flexibility in Hong Kong Chinese Adults: A Controlled Clinical Trial.
Evidence-based Complementary and Alternative Medicine : eCAM.
2015;2015:958727. doi:10.1155/2015/958727.

4. Ulger O, Yagli NV. Effects of yoga on balance and gait properties in
women with musculoskeletal problems: a pilot study. Complement Ther
Clin Pract. 2011;17(1):13–15. doi: 10.1016/j.ctcp.2010.06.006.

5. B. Donahoe-Fillmore, M. Holdash, C. Moore, J. Robertson. The effect of
yoga postures on balance, coordination and flexibility in typically
developing children. Pediatric Physical Therapy: April 2004 - Volume 16
- Issue 1 - p 51. doi: 10.1097/01.PEP.0000115221.39160.D5.

6. Abel AN, Lloyd LK, Williams JS. The effects of regular yoga practice on
pulmonary function in healthy individuals: A literature review. J Altern
Complement Med. 2013;19:185–90.

7. Maheshkumar Kuppusamy, K Dilara, P Ravishankar, and A Julius.
Effect of Bhrāmarī Prāṇāyāma Practice on Pulmonary Function in
Healthy Adolescents: A Randomized Control Study. Anc Sci Life. 2017
Apr-Jun; 36(4): 196–199.

8. Yadav RK, Das S. Effect of yogic practice on pulmonary functions in
young females. I ndian J Physiol Pharmacol. 2001 Oct;45(4):493-6.

9. Telles S, Singh N, Balkrishna A. Metabolic and Ventilatory Changes During and After High-Frequency Yoga Breathing. Medical Science Monitor Basic Research. 2015;21:161-171. doi:10.12659/MSMBR.894945.

10. Mandanmohan, Jatiya L, Udupa K, Bhavanani AB. Effect of yoga training on handgrip, respiratory pressures and pulmonary function. Indian J Physiol Pharmacol. 2003 Oct;47(4):387-92.

11. Brook R.D., Appel L.J., Rubenfire M. Beyond medications and diet. Alternative approaches to lowering blood pressure. A Scientific Statement from American Heart Association. Hypertension. 2013;61:1360–1363.

12. Sivasankaran S, Pollard-Quintner S, Sachdeva R, Pugeda J, Hoq SM, Zarich SW. The effect of a six-week program of yoga and meditation on brachial artery reactivity: do psychosocial interventions affect vascular tone? Clin Cardiol. 2006 Sep;29(9):393-8.

13. Pal A, Srivastava N, Tiwari S, Verma NS, Narain VS, Agrawal GG, Natu SM, Kumar K. Effect of yogic practices on lipid profile and body fat composition in patients of coronary artery disease. Complement Ther Med. 2011;19:122–127.

14. Raghuram N, Parachuri VR, Swarnagowri MV, et al. Yoga based cardiac rehabilitation after coronary artery bypass surgery: One-year results on LVEF, lipid profile and psychological states – A randomized controlled study. Indian Heart Journal. 2014;66(5):490-502. doi:10.1016/j.ihj.2014.08.007.

15. Miles SC, Chun-Chung C, Hsin-Fu L, Hunter SD, Dhindsa M, Nualnim N, Tanaka H. Arterial blood pressure and cardiovascular responses to yoga practice. Altern Ther Health Med. 2013 Jan-Feb;19(1):38-45.

16. Tyagi A, Cohen M. Yoga and heart rate variability: A comprehensive review of the literature. International Journal of Yoga. 2016;9(2):97-113. doi:10.4103/0973-6131.183712.

17. Manchanda S.C., Narang R., Reddy K.S. Retardation of coronary atherosclerosis with yoga lifestyle intervention. J Assoc Physicians India. 2000;48:687–694.

18. Kamei T, Toriumi Y, Kimura H, Ohno S, Kumano H, Kimura K. Decrease in serum cortisol during yoga exercise is correlated with alpha wave activation. Percept Mot Skills. 2000;90(3 Pt 1):1027–1032.

19. Ross A, Thomas S. The health benefits of yoga and exercise: a review of comparison studies. J Altern Complement Med. 2010;16(1):3–12.

20. Streeter CC, Jensen JE, Perlmutter RM, Cabral HJ, Tian H, Terhune DB, Ciraulo DA, Renshaw PF. Yoga asana sessions increase brain GABA levels: a pilot study. J Altern Complement Med. 2007;13(4):419–426. doi: 10.1089/acm.2007.6338.

21. Streeter CC, Whitfield TH, Owen L, et al. Effects of yoga versus walking on mood, anxiety, and brain GABA levels: a randomized controlled MRS study. J Altern Complement Med. 2010;16(11):1145–1152.

22. Streeter CC, Gerbarg PL, Saper RB, et al. Effects of yoga on the autonomic nervous system, gamma-aminobutyric-acid, and allostasis in epilepsy, depression, and post-traumatic stress disorder. Med Hypotheses. 2012;78(5):571–579.

23. Pal R, Singh SN, Chatterjee A, Saha M. Age-related changes in cardiovascular system, autonomic functions, and levels of BDNF of

healthy active males: role of yogic practice. Age. 2014;36(4):9683. doi:10.1007/s11357-014-9683-7.

24. Schultz W. Getting formal with dopamine and reward. Neuron. 2002;36(2):241–263.

25. Jayaram N, Varambally S, Behere RV, et al. Effect of yoga therapy on plasma oxytocin and facial emotion recognition deficits in patients of schizophrenia. Indian Journal of Psychiatry. 2013;55(Suppl 3): S409-S413. doi:10.4103/0019-5545.116318.

26. Froeliger B, Garland EL, McClernon FJ. Yoga Meditation Practitioners Exhibit Greater Gray Matter Volume and Fewer Reported Cognitive Failures: Results of a Preliminary Voxel-Based Morphometric Analysis. Evidence-based Complementary and Alternative Medicine: eCAM. 2012;2012:821307. doi:10.1155/2012/821307.

27. Afonso RF, Balardin JB, Lazar S, et al. Greater Cortical Thickness in Elderly Female Yoga Practitioners—A Cross-Sectional Study. Frontiers in Aging Neuroscience. 2017;9:201. doi:10.3389/fnagi.2017.00201.

28. Hariprasad VR, Varambally S, Shivakumar V, Kalmady SV, Venkatasubramanian G, Gangadhar BN. Yoga increases the volume of the hippocampus in elderly subjects. Indian Journal of Psychiatry. 2013;55(Suppl 3): S394-S396. doi:10.4103/0019-5545.116309.

29. Hölzel BK, Carmody J, Evans KC, et al. Stress reduction correlates with structural changes in the amygdala. Social Cognitive and Affective Neuroscience. 2010;5(1):11-17. doi:10.1093/scan/nsp034.

30. Gard T, Hölzel BK, Lazar SW. The potential effects of meditation on age-related cognitive decline: a systematic review. Annals of the New York Academy of Sciences. 2014;1307:89-103. doi:10.1111/nyas.12348.

31. Cahn BR, Goodman MS, Peterson CT, Maturi R, Mills PJ. Yoga, Meditation and Mind-Body Health: Increased BDNF, Cortisol Awakening Response, and Altered Inflammatory Marker Expression after a 3-Month Yoga and Meditation Retreat. Frontiers in Human Neuroscience. 2017;11:315. doi:10.3389/fnhum.2017.00315.

32. Tooley GA, Armstrong SM, Norman TR, Sali A. Acute increases in Night-time plasma melatonin levels following a period of mediatation. Biol Psychol. 2000;53:69–78.

33. Cahn BR, Goodman MS, Peterson CT, Maturi R, Mills PJ. Yoga, Meditation and Mind-Body Health: Increased BDNF, Cortisol Awakening Response, and Altered Inflammatory Marker Expression after a 3-Month Yoga and Meditation Retreat. Frontiers in Human Neuroscience. 2017;11:315. doi:10.3389/fnhum.2017.00315.

34. Zeidan F, Martucci KT, Kraft RA, McHaffie JG, Coghill RC. Neural correlates of mindfulness meditation-related anxiety relief. Social Cognitive and Affective Neuroscience. 2014;9(6):751-759. doi:10.1093/scan/nst041.

35. Newberg A, Alavi A, Baime M, Pourdehnad M, Santanna J, d'Aquili E. The measurement of regional cerebral blood flow during the complex cognitive task of meditation: a preliminary SPECT study. Psychiatry Res. 2001;106(2):113–22.

36. Jim Lagopoulos, Jian Xu, Inge Rasmussen, Alexandra Vik, Gin S. Malhi, Carl F. Eliassen, Ingrid E. Arntsen, Jardar G. Sæther, Stig Hollup, Are Holen, Svend Davanger, and Øyvind Ellingsen. Increased theta and alpha EEG activity during nondirective meditation. The Journal of

Alternative and Complementary Medicine. November 2009, 15(11): 1187-1192.

37. Pal R, Singh SN, Chatterjee A, Saha M. Age-related changes in cardiovascular system, autonomic functions, and levels of BDNF of healthy active males: role of yogic practice. Age. 2014;36(4):9683. doi:10.1007/s11357-014-9683-7.

38. Khattab K, Khattab AA, Ortak J, Richardt G, Bonnemeier H. Iyengar yoga increases cardiac parasympathetic nervous modulation among healthy yoga practitioners. Evid Based Complement Alternat Med. 2007;4:511–7.

39. Vinay A, Venkatesh D, Ambarish V. Impact of short-term practice of yoga on heart rate variability. International Journal of Yoga. 2016;9(1):62-66. doi:10.4103/0973-6131.171714.

40. Bharshankar JR, Mandape AD, Phatak MS, Bharshankar RN. Autonomic Functions in Raja-yoga Meditators. Indian J Physiol Pharmacol. 2015 Oct-Dec;59(4):396-401.

41. Bhaskar L, Kharya C, Deepak KK, Kochupillai V. Assessment of Cardiac Autonomic Tone Following Long Sudarshan Kriya Yoga in Art of Living Practitioners. J Altern Complement Med. 2017 Sep;23(9):705-712. doi: 10.1089/acm.2016.0391. Epub 2017 Jul 10.

42. Pullen PR, Nagamia SH, Mehta PK, Thompson WR, Benardot D, Hammoud R, et al. Effects of yoga on inflammation and exercise capacity in patients with chronic heart failure. J Card Fail. 2008;14(5):407–13.

43. Bower JE, Irwin MR. Mind-body therapies and control of inflammatory biology: A descriptive review. Brain, behavior, and immunity. 2016;51:1-11.

44. Cahn BR, Goodman MS, Peterson CT, Maturi R, Mills PJ. Yoga, Meditation and Mind-Body Health: Increased BDNF, Cortisol Awakening Response, and Altered Inflammatory Marker Expression after a 3-Month Yoga and Meditation Retreat. Frontiers in Human Neuroscience. 2017;11:315. doi:10.3389/fnhum.2017.00315.

45. Rodolfo Paoletti, Antonio M. Gotto, David P. Hajjar. Inflammation in Atherosclerosis and Implications for Therapy. Circulation. 2004;109:III-20-III-26.

46. Coussens LM, Werb Z. Inflammation and cancer. Nature. 2002;420(6917):860-867. doi:10.1038/nature01322.

47. Villemure C, Čeko M, Cotton VA, Bushnell MC. Insular Cortex Mediates Increased Pain Tolerance in Yoga Practitioners. Cerebral Cortex (New York, NY). 2014;24(10):2732-2740. doi:10.1093/cercor/bht124.

48. Gopal A, Mondal S, Gandhi A, Arora S, Bhattacharjee J. Effect of integrated yoga practices on immune responses in examination stress - A preliminary study. Int J Yoga. 2011;4:26–32.

49. Woodyard C. Exploring the therapeutic effects of yoga and its ability to increase quality of life. International Journal of Yoga. 2011;4(2):49-54. doi:10.4103/0973-6131.85485.

50. Stussman BJ, Black LI, Barnes PM, Clarke TC, Nahin RL. Wellness-related use of common complementary health approaches among adults: United States, 2012. National health statistics reports; no 85. Hyattsville, MD: National Center for Health Statistics. 2015.

51. Agarwal SK. Evidence based health benefits of yoga. Book. 2018. Available at Amazon.
52. https://health.gov/paguidelines/pdf/paguide.pdf - accessed 1/26/18.
53. Jetté M, Sidney K, Blümchen G. Metabolic equivalents (METS) in exercise testing, exercise prescription, and evaluation of functional capacity. Clin Cardiol. 1990 Aug;13(8):555-65.
54. https://health.gov/paguidelines/guidelines/appendix1.aspx - accessed 1/27/18.
55. Larson-Meyer DE. A Systematic Review of the Energy Cost and Metabolic Intensity of Yoga. Med Sci Sports Exerc. 2016 Aug;48(8):1558-69. doi: 10.1249/MSS.0000000000000922.
56. Boyd CN, Lannan SM, Zuhl MN, Mora-Rodriguez R, Nelson RK. Objective and subjective measures of exercise intensity during thermo-neutral and hot yoga. Appl Physiol Nutr Metab. 2017 Nov 23. doi: 10.1139/apnm-2017-0495.
57. Hagins M, Moore W, Rundle A. Does practicing hatha yoga satisfy recommendations for intensity of physical activity which improves and maintains health and cardiovascular fitness? BMC Complementary and Alternative Medicine. 2007;7:40. doi:10.1186/1472-6882-7-40.
58. Melanie Potiaumpai, Maria Carolina Massoni Martins, Roberto Rodriguez, Kiersten Mooney, Joseph F. Signorile. Differences in energy expenditure during high-speed versus standard-speed yoga: A randomized sequence crossover trial. Complementary Therapies in Medicine, Volume 29, December 2016, Pages 169-174.
59. Satish V, Rao RM, Manjunath NK, Amritanshu R, Vivek U, Shreeganesh HR, Deepashree S. Yoga versus physical exercise for cardio-respiratory fitness in adolescent school children: a randomized controlled trial. Int J Adolesc Med Health. 2018 Jan 25. pii: /j/ijamh.ahead-of-print/ijamh-2017-0154.
60. Boyd CN, Lannan SM, Zuhl MN, Mora-Rodriguez R, Nelson RK. Objective and subjective measures of exercise intensity during thermo-neutral and hot yoga. Appl Physiol Nutr Metab. 2017 Nov 23. doi: 10.1139/apnm-2017-0495.
61. Sinha B, Ray US, Pathak A, Selvamurthy W. Energy cost and cardiorespiratory changes during the practice of surya namaskar. Indian J Physiol Pharmacol. 2004;48:184–90.
62. Cramer H, Lauche R, Dobos G. Characteristics of randomized controlled trials of yoga: a bibliometric analysis. BMC Complementary and Alternative Medicine. 2014;14:328. doi:10.1186/1472-6882-14-328.
63. Feuerstein G. The Yoga Tradition. Prescott: Hohm Press; 1998.; De Michaelis E. A History of Modern Yoga: Patanjali and Western Esotericism. London, UK: Continuum International Publishing Group; 2005.
64. Woodyard C. Exploring the therapeutic effects of yoga and its ability to increase quality of life. Intern J Yoga 2011;4:49–54.
65. Agarwal SK. Evidence Based Therapeutic Effects of Yoga. Book. 2018. Available at Amazon.

WHAT IS YOGA

1.   https://nccih.nih.gov/health/yoga.
2.   Barnes P, Bloom B, Nahin R. Complementary and alternative medicine use among adults and children: United States, 2007. Natl Health Stat Report. 2008. December 10;(12):1–23.
3.   Larson-Meyer DE. A Systematic Review of the Energy Cost and Metabolic Intensity of Yoga. Med Sci Sports Exerc. 2016 Aug;48(8):1558-69. doi: 10.1249/MSS.0000000000000922.
4.   NHS . Your health, your choices. A guide to yoga. 2013.
5.   https: //www.usatoday.com/story/opinion/2013/05/18/yoga-religion-column/2158377/ (accessed 1/2/18).
6.   Keosaian JE, Lemaster CM, Dresner D, et al. "We're All in This Together": A Qualitative Study of Predominantly Low Income Minority Participants in a Yoga Trial for Chronic Low Back Pain. Complementary therapies in medicine. 2016;24:34-39. doi:10.1016/j.ctim.2015.11.007.
7.   Firestone KA, Carson JW, Mist SD, Carson KM, Jones KD. Interest In Yoga Among Fibromyalgia Patients: An International Internet Survey. International journal of yoga therapy. 2014;24:117-124.
8.   Berger DL, Silver EJ, Stein REK. Effects of yoga on inner-city children's well-being: a pilot study. Alternative Therapies in Health and Medicine. 2009;15(5):36–42.
9.   Curtis K, Hitzig SL, Bechsgaard G, et al. Evaluation of a specialized yoga program for persons with a spinal cord injury: a pilot randomized controlled trial. Journal of Pain Research. 2017;10:999-1017. doi:10.2147/JPR.S130530.
10. Balasubramaniam M., Telles S., Doraiswamy P. M. (2012). Yoga on our minds: a systematic review of yoga for neuropsychiatric disorders. Front. Psychiatry 3:117. 10.3389/fpsyt.2012.00117.
11. Rector K, Vilardaga R, Lansky L, et al. Design and Real-World Evaluation of Eyes-Free Yoga: An Exergame for Blind and Low-Vision Exercise. ACM transactions on accessible computing. 2017;9(4):12. doi:10.1145/3022729.
12. https://www.livestrong.com/article/394069-do-you-need-to-use-a-yoga-mat - accessed 12/5/17.
13. Tew GA, Howsam J, Hardy M, Bissell L. Adapted yoga to improve physical function and health-related quality of life in physically-inactive older adults: a randomised controlled pilot trial. BMC Geriatrics. 2017;17:131.
14. Cramer H, Krucoff C, Dobos G. Adverse events associated with yoga: a systematic review of published case reports and case series. PLoS One. 2013;8(10):e75515. doi: 10.1371/journal.pone.0075515.
15. Cheema BS, Marshall PW, Chang D, Colagiuri B, Machliss B. Effect of an office worksite-based yoga program on heart rate variability: A randomized controlled trial. BMC Public Health. 2011;11:578. doi:10.1186/1471-2458-11-578.
16. Berger DL, Silver EJ, Stein RE. Effects of yoga on inner-city children's well-being: a pilot study. Altern Ther Health Med. 2009 Sep-Oct;15(5):36-42.

17. Chen KM, Fan JT, Wang HH, Wu SJ, Li CH, Lin HS. Silver yoga exercises improved physical fitness of transitional frail elders. Nurs Res. 2010 Sep-Oct;59(5):364-70. doi: 10.1097/NNR.0b013e3181ef37d5.

18. Flegal K, Kishiyama S, Zajdel D, Haas M, Oken B. Adherence to yoga and exercise interventions in a 6-month clinical trial. BMC Complementary and Alternative Medicine. 2007;7:37. doi:10.1186/1472-6882-7-37.

19. Tew GA, Howsam J, Hardy M, Bissell L. Adapted yoga to improve physical function and health-related quality of life in physically-inactive older adults: a randomised controlled pilot trial. BMC Geriatrics. 2017;17:131. doi:10.1186/s12877-017-0520-6.

20. Findorff MJ, Wyman JF, Gross CR. Predictors of Long-term Exercise Adherence in a Community-Based Sample of Older Women. Journal of Women's Health. 2009;18(11):1769-1776. doi:10.1089/jwh.2008.1265.

21. Mishra SK, Singh P, Bunch SJ, Zhang R. The therapeutic value of yoga in neurological disorders. Annals of Indian Academy of Neurology. 2012;15(4):247-254. doi:10.4103/0972-2327.104328.

22. Findorff MJ, Wyman JF, Gross CR. Predictors of Long-term Exercise Adherence in a Community-Based Sample of Older Women. Journal of Women's Health. 2009;18(11):1769-1776. doi:10.1089/jwh.2008.1265.

23. Agarwal SK. Evidence Based Therapeutic Effects of Yoga. 2017.Available at: https://www.amazon.com/Evidence-Based-Therapeutic-Effects-Yoga/dp/1983936367/ref=sr_1_3?s=books&ie=UTF8&qid=1517713441 &sr=1-3&keywords=agarwal+shashi+k

24. National Center for Complementary and Alternative Medicine. Yoga for Health: Side Effects and Risks. Online document at: http://nccam.nih.gov/health/yoga/introduction.htm#hed3 Accessed January30, 2014.

25. https://www.yogajournal.com/lifestyle/8-travel-yoga-poses-work-small-spaces - accessed 12/15/17.

26. Vyavahare SV. Yoga for jail inmates. Proceedings of the 1st International Conference on Frontiers in Yoga Research and Applications; December 1991; Bangalore, India. VKYRF.

27. Ross A, Friedmann E, Bevans M, Thomas S. National Survey of Yoga Practitioners: Mental and Physical Health Benefits. Complementary therapies in medicine. 13;21(4):313-323. doi:10.1016/j.ctim.2013.04.001.

28. Birdee GS, Ayala SG, Wallston KA. Cross-sectional analysis of health-related quality of life and elements of yoga practice. BMC Complementary and Alternative Medicine. 2017;17:83. doi:10.1186/s12906-017-1599-1.

MEDITATION (DHYANA)

1. Northoff G. Heinzel A. de Greck M. Bermpohl F. Dobrowolny H. Panksepp J. (2006). Self-referential processing in our brain—a meta-analysis of imaging studies on the self. Neuroimage, 31 (1), 440 – 57.

2. Denny B.T. Kober H. Wager T.D. Ochsner K.N. (2012). A meta-analysis of functional neuroimaging studies of self-and other judgments reveals a

spatial gradient for mentalizing in medial prefrontal cortex. Journal of Cognitive Neuroscience, 24 (8), 1742 – 52.

3. Bartra O. McGuire J.T. Kable J.W. (2013). The valuation system: a coordinate-based meta-analysis of {BOLD} fMRI experiments examining neural correlates of subjective value. NeuroImage, 76, 412 – 27.

4. Dfarhud D, Malmir M, Khanahmadi M. "Happiness & Health: The Biological Factors- Systematic Review Article." Iranian Journal of Public Health 43.11 (2014): 1468–1477.)

ADVERSE EFFECTS OF YOGA

1. https://nccih.nih.gov/research/statistics/2007/camsurvey_fs1.htm - accessed 2/23/18.

2. https://nccih.nih.gov/health/yoga - accessed 2/13/18.

3. Ross A, Friedmann E, Bevans M, Thomas S. National Survey of Yoga Practitioners: Mental and Physical Health Benefits. Complementary therapies in medicine. 2013;21(4):313-323. doi:10.1016/j.ctim.2013.04.001.

4. Agarwal SK. Evidence Based Therapeutic Effects of Yoga. 2017.Available at: https://www.amazon.com/Evidence-Based-Therapeutic-Effects-Yoga/dp/1983936367/ref=sr_1_3?s=books&ie=UTF8&qid=1517713441&sr=1-3&keywords=agarwal+shashi+k.

5. Swain TA, McGwin G. Yoga-Related Injuries in the United States From 2001 to 2014. Orthopaedic Journal of Sports Medicine. 2016;4(11):2325967116671703. doi:10.1177/2325967116671703.

6. Fishman LM, Saltonstall E, Genis S. Yoga therapy in practice; understanding and preventing yoga injuries. Int J Yoga Ther. 2009;19:123–128.

7. Cowen VS. Functional fitness improvements after a worksite-based yoga initiative. J Bodyw Mov Ther. 2010;14(1):50–4. doi: 10.1016/j.jbmt.2009.02.006.

8. Takeno M, Shimizu Y, Nakamura S. A case of femoral shaft fracture occurring during stretching exercise. J Clinical Sports Med. 1986;3(1):75–8.

9. Patel SC, Parker DA. Isolated rupture of the lateral collateral ligament during yoga practice: a case report. J Orthop Surg (Hong Kong) 2008;16(3):378–80.

10. Shah NJ, Shah UN. Central retinal vein occlusion following Sirsasana (headstand posture) Indian J Ophthalmol. 2009;57(1):69–70. doi: 10.4103/0301-4738.44496.

11. Johnson DB, Tierney MJ, Sadighi PJ. Kapalabhati pranayama: breath of fire or cause of pneumothorax? A case report. Chest. 2004;125(5):1951–2.

12. Holton MK, Barry AE. Do side-effects/injuries from yoga practice result in discontinued use? Results of a national survey. Int J Yoga. 2014;7:152–154

12.APPENDIX

YOGA SEQUENCE I – 60 POSES

TOTAL TIME APPROXIMATELY 45 MINUTES

(Poses 30 minutes, breathing exercises 10 minutes and meditation 5 minutes)

Poses are entered into either during inhalation or exhalation.

Breathing Time each pose: Inhalation or entering or leaving pose: 5 seconds; normal breathing during hold phase of pose: 10 seconds; exhalation on entering or leaving pose: 5 seconds. Time in between poses: 5-10 seconds. These are approximates – use timings that are convenient to you.

Meditation: normal breathing

POSES (Asanas):

Time: approximately 30 minutes

STANDING POSES

1. Mountain Pose
2. Upward Salute
3. Standing half forward bend
4. Modified Mountain Pose
5. Crescent Moon in Mountain Pose
6. Deep Forward Bend
7. Right Leg Forward Bend Both Hands
8. Left Leg Forward Bend Both Hands
9. Wide Legged Mountain Pose
10. Both Hands to Right Big Toe Pose; With left hand up / revolve to right hand up
11. Both Hands to Left Big Toe Pose; With right hand up / revolve to left hand up
12. Crescent Moon in Wide Legged Mountain Pose
13. Forward Bend with palms on floor
14. Right Side Bend in Wide Legged Mountain Pose
15. Left Side Bend in Wide Legged Mountain Pose
16. Warrior I: Right Foot Forward - Right Knee Bent

17. Forward High Lunge in Warrior I Right Foot Forward - Right Knee Bent
18. Reverse Warrior with Right Foot Forward - Right Knee Bent
19. Warrior I: Left Foot Forward - Left Knee Bent
20. Forward High Lunge in Warrior I: Left Foot Forward - Left Knee Bent
21. Reverse Warrior with Left Foot Forward
22. Warrior II with Right Knee Bent - Twist Right and hold and then Left
23. Warrior II with Left Knee Bent - Twist Left and hold and then Right
24. Standing Chair

KNEELING/SITTING POSES:

25. Garland
26. Hero Pose
27. Easy Pose
28. Butterfly
29. Staff Pose
30. Half Bound Forward Bend - Right Leg Straight
31. Half Bound Forward Bend - Left Leg Straight
32. Thunderbolt Pose
33. Crescent Moon in Hero Pose
34. Child Pose
35. Extended Puppy Pose
36. Standing Thunderbolt
37. Gate Latch: Right Leg Extended
38. Gate Latch: Left Leg Extended
39. Downward Facing Dog
40. Low Lunge: Lizard: Right Knee Front and Bent
41. Low Lunge: Lizard: Left Knee Front and Bent

LYING FACE DOWN POSES

42. Sphynx
43. Dolphin Plank
44. Cobra
45. Upward Facing Dog
46. Downward Facing Plank
47. Locust
48. Bow
49. Reclining Buddha: Right Side
50. Side Plank: Right Side
51. Reclining Buddha: Left Side

52. Side Plank: Left Side

LYING FACE UP POSES

53. Corpse Pose
54. Boat - Full Boat
55. Happy Baby Pose
56. Wind Relief Pose
57. Bridge Pose
58. Upward Plank
59. Supine Spinal Twist Right Side
60. Supine Spinal Twist Left Side

Final: Corpse Pose to supine stretch and back to corpse pose.

BREATHING EXERCISES: (in Corpse Pose or Easy Pose)

Time: 10 minutes

After the asanas. relax in corpse position with silk breath for one minute or so. Then proceed to the breathing exercises.

1. Complete breath without Locks: One Cycle = 20 seconds: Inhalation 5 seconds; Hold 5 seconds; Exhalation 5 seconds; Hold 5 seconds. Do 6 cycles. (2 minutes)
2. Complete breath with locks: One Cycle = 20 seconds: Inhalation 5 seconds; Hold 5 seconds; Exhalation 5 seconds; Hold with locks 5 seconds. Do 6 cycles. (2 minutes)
3. Alternate Nostril Breathing: One Cycle = 40 seconds: Inhale Left nostril 5 seconds; Hold 5 seconds; Exhale Right Nostril 5 seconds; Hold for 5 seconds; Inhale Right Nostril 5 seconds; Hold 5 seconds; Exhale Left Nostril 5 seconds; Hold 5 seconds. Do 6 cycles. (4 minutes)
4. Core massaging breath. (1 minute)

Relax with silk breath for one minute before proceeding to the meditation sequence.

MEDITATION: (in Easy or Corpse Pose)

Time: 5 minutes do any one or all of these:

1. Silk breath meditation
2. Mantra meditation
3. Thoughtless meditation

4. Meditative visualization
5. Meditative affirmations

Relax in corpse pose as needed.

YOGA SEQUENCE II – 90 POSES

TOTAL TIME APPROXIMATELY 60-75 MINUTES

(Poses 45 minutes, breathing exercises 15 minutes and meditation 20 minutes – timings are approximate and can be altered depending upon your convenience)

POSES (Asanas):

Time: approximately 45 minutes

Poses are entered into either during inhalation or exhalation. Breathing time each pose: Inhalation or entering or leaving pose: 5 seconds; normal breathing during hold phase of pose: 10 seconds; exhalation on entering or leaving pose: 5 seconds. Time in between poses: 5-10 seconds.

STANDING POSES

1. Mountain Pose
2. Upward Salute
3. Swaying Tree Pose - Right Side
4. Swaying Tree Pose - Left Side
5. Tree Pose - Right leg up
6. Tree Pose - Left leg up
7. Standing half forward bend Extended Hand-To-Big-Toe Pose – Right leg up
8. Extended Hand-To-Big-Toe Pose – Left leg up
9. Modified Mountain Pose
10. Crescent Moon in Mountain Pose
11. Deep Forward Bend
12. Right Leg Forward Bend Both Hands
13. Left Leg Forward Bend Both Hands
14. Wide Legged Mountain Pose
15. Both Hands to Right Big Toe Pose; With left hand up / revolve to right hand up
16. Both Hands to Left Big Toe Pose; With right hand up / revolve to left hand up
17. Crescent Moon in Wide Legged Mountain Pose
18. Forward Bend with palms on floor

19. Wide-Legged Standing Forward Fold with head on floor
20. Right Side Bend in Wide Legged Mountain Pose
21. Balancing star – Right arm down
22. Left Side Bend in Wide Legged Mountain Pose
23. Balancing star – Left arm down
24. Warrior I: Right Foot Forward - Right Knee Bent
25. Forward High Lunge in Warrior I Right Foot Forward - Right Knee Bent
26. Reverse Warrior with Right Foot Forward - Right Knee Bent
27. Extended Side Angle Pose – Right leg bent
28. Revolved Side Angle Pose – Right leg bent
29. Warrior I: Left Foot Forward - Left Knee Bent
30. Forward High Lunge in Warrior I: Left Foot Forward - Left Knee Bent
31. Reverse Warrior with Left Foot Forward
32. Extended Side Angle Pose – Left leg bent
33. Revolved Side Angle Pose – Left leg bent
34. Warrior II with Right Knee Bent - Twist Right and hold then Left
35. Warrior II with Left Knee Bent - Twist Left and hold and then Right
36. Standing Chair

KNEELING/SITTING POSES:

37. Garland Pose
38. Hero Pose
39. Half Spinal Twist Pose – Right side
40. Half Spinal Twist Pose – Left side
41. Easy Pose
42. Butterfly Pose
43. Staff Pose
44. Half Bound Forward Bend - Right Leg Straight
45. Half Bound Forward Bend - Left Leg Straight
46. Revolved Head to Knee Pose – Right leg
47. Revolved Head to Knee Pose – Left leg
48. Thunderbolt Pose
49. Crescent Moon in Hero Pose
50. Child Pose
51. Extended Puppy Pose
52. Standing Thunderbolt
53. Camel Pose
54. Gate Latch: Right Leg Extended
55. Gate Latch: Left Leg Extended
56. Downward Facing Dog
57. Low Lunge: Lizard: Right Knee Front and Bent
58. Modified low lung – Right knee Bent

59. Low Lunge: Lizard: Left Knee Front and Bent
60. Modified low lung – Left knee Bent
61. Dolphin Pose
62. Reverse Corpse Pose

LYING FACE DOWN POSES

63. Sphynx
64. Dolphin Plank
65. Cobra
66. Upward Facing Dog
67. Downward Facing Plank
68. Four Limbed Staff Pose
69. Cat Pose
70. Cow Pose
71. Locust Pose
72. Bow Pose
73. Reclining Buddha: Right side
74. Reclining Buddha Right side with Left leg up
75. Side Plank: Right Side
76. Reclining Buddha: Left Side
77. Reclining Buddha Left side with Right leg up
78. Side Plank: Left Side

LYING FACE UP POSES

79. Corpse Pose
80. Boat - Full Boat Pose
81. Fish Pose
82. Happy Baby Pose
83. Wind Relief Pose
84. Bridge Pose
85. Upward Plank
86. Reclining Bound Angle Pose
87. Supine Spinal Twist Right Side
88. Supine Spinal Twist Left Side
89. Shoulder Stand
90. Final: Corpse Pose to supine stretch and back to corpse pose.

BREATHING EXERCISES: (in Corpse Pose or Easy Pose)

Time: 15 minutes

Complete breath with holds: 6 cycles: 2 minutes
2. Complete breath with locks: 6 cycles: 2 minutes

3. Alternate nostril breathing: 6 cycles: 4 minutes
4. Ujjayi breathing: 12 cycles: 2 minutes
5. Chakra breathing: 3 minutes
6. Core massaging breathing: 12 breaths: 1 minute
7. Relaxed silk breath: 1 minute

MEDITATION: (in Easy or Corpse Pose)

Time: 20 minutes
Do any one or all of these:

- Silk breath meditation
- Mantra meditation
- Thoughtless meditation
- Chakra meditation
- Mindfulness
- Meditative visualization
- Meditative affirmations

Relax in corpse pose as needed.

*"Breathing in, I calm body and mind. Breathing out, I smile.
Dwelling in the present moment I know this is the only moment."*

Nhat Hanh

13. RESOURCES

Books

* The Yoga Bible. Christina Brown. Walking Stick Press
* The Women's Health Big Book of Yoga: The Essential Guide to Complete Mind/Body Fitness. Kathryn Budig. Rodale Books
* Light on Yoga. B.K.S. Iyengar. Harper Collins Publishers
* Yoga as Medicine: The Yogic Prescription for Health and Healing. Timothy Mccall. Bantam.
* Anatomy of Hatha Yoga: A Manual for Students, Teachers, and Practitioners. H. David Coulter. Body and Breath
* Evidence Based Health Benefits of Yoga. Shashi K. Agarwal, MD. CreateSpace Independent Publishing (Amazon)
* The Yoga Sutras of Patanjali. Integral Yoga Publications
* Evidence Based Therapeutic Effects of Yoga. Shashi K. Agarwal, MD. CreateSpace Independent Publishing (Amazon)

Professional Yoga Associations

* iayt.org (International Association of Yoga Therapists)
* yogaalliance.org (Yoga Alliance)

Non-professional Magazines

* Australian Yoga Life
* Integral Yoga Magazine
* LA Yoga
* OM Yoga & Lifestyle Magazine
* Yoga Journal

ALSO BY AUTHOR

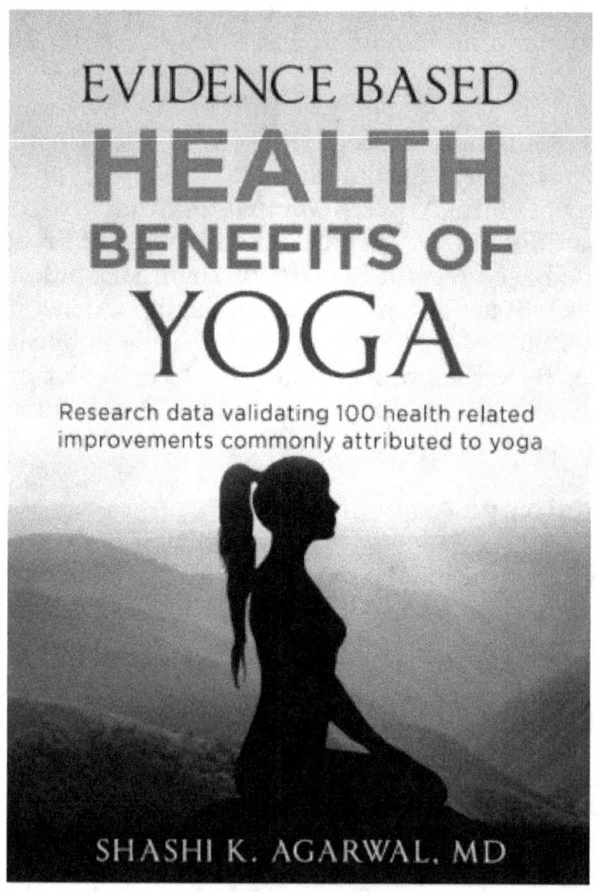

478 pages $24.99

Available at amazon.com

ALSO BY AUTHOR

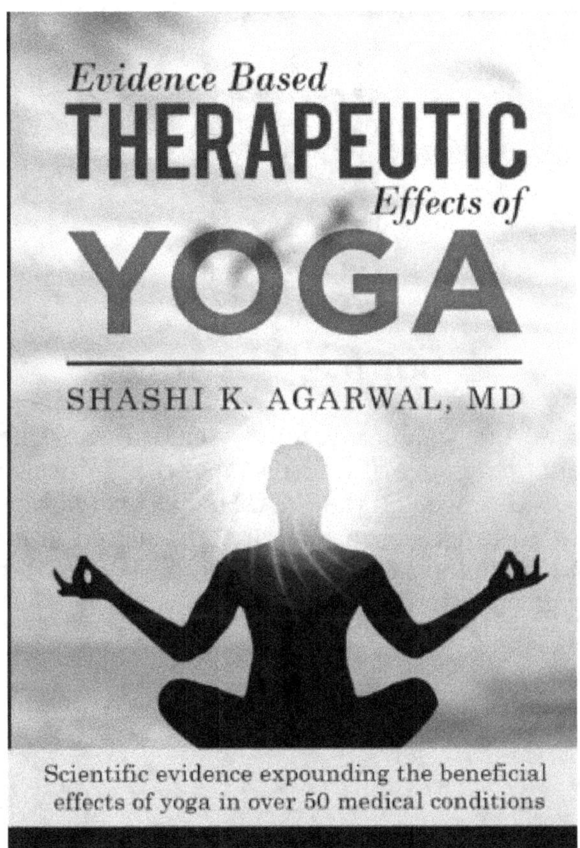

254 Pages $15.99

Available at amazon.com

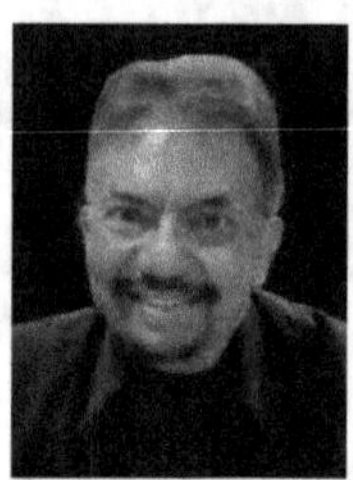

ABOUT THE AUTHOR

Dr. Shashi K. Agarwal has presented scientific abstracts on the health benefits of yoga at international conferences in India, Glasgow, UK, France and the USA. He has also published yoga related scientific articles in several national and international journals and given talks on the evidence-based health benefits of yoga at several national meetings in the USA.